ADHD

Amazing Activities to Help Children Self-regulate, Focus, and Succeed

(Proven Adhd Tips for Dealing With Attention Deficit Disorder and Hyperactive Kids)

Thomas Dejesus

Published by Rob Miles

© **Thomas Dejesus**

All Rights Reserved

Adhd: Amazing Activities to Help Children Self-regulate, Focus, and Succeed (Proven Adhd Tips for Dealing With Attention Deficit Disorder and Hyperactive Kids)

ISBN 978-1-990084-14-0

All rights reserved. No part of this guide may be reproduced in any form without permission in writing from the publisher except in the case of brief quotations embodied in critical articles or reviews.
Legal & Disclaimer

The information contained in this book is not designed to replace or take the place of any form of medicine or professional medical advice. The information in this book has been provided for educational and entertainment purposes only.

The information contained in this book has been compiled from sources deemed reliable, and it is accurate to the best of the Author's knowledge; however, the Author cannot guarantee its accuracy and validity and cannot be held liable for any errors or omissions. Changes are periodically made to this book. You must consult your doctor or get professional medical advice before using any of the suggested remedies, techniques, or information in this book.

Upon using the information contained in this book, you agree to hold harmless the Author from and against any damages, costs, and expenses, including any legal fees potentially resulting from the application of any of the information provided by this guide. This disclaimer applies to any damages or injury caused by the use and application, whether directly or indirectly, of any advice or information presented, whether for breach of contract, tort, negligence, personal injury, criminal intent, or under any other cause of action.

You agree to accept all risks of using the information presented inside this book. You need to consult a professional medical practitioner in order to ensure you are both able and healthy enough to participate in this program.

Table of Contents

INTRODUCTION 1

CHAPTER 1: WHAT PARENTS NEED TO KNOW 3

CHAPTER 2: ADHD, ITS SIGNS, SYMPTOMS AND TREATMENT 17

CHAPTER 3: WHAT IS ADHD? 28

CHAPTER 4: SCIENCE AND REAL LIFE 40

CHAPTER 5: THE INTRODUCTION OF BENZEDRINE 46

CHAPTER 6: ADD: HOW IS IT DIFFERENT FROM ADHD? ... 56

CHAPTER 7: WHAT THE HECK IS ADHD ANYWAYS? 68

CHAPTER 8: PARENTING IN PUBLIC 72

CHAPTER 9: CAUSES OF ADHD 76

CHAPTER 10: ALL ABOUT ADHD: CAUSES, TYPES, AND RISK FACTORS 81

CHAPTER 11: ADHD FOR PARENTS 91

CHAPTER 12: ADULT ADHD SYMPTOMS - WHICH TYPE OF ADHD ARE YOU FACING? 109

CHAPTER 13: ADHD IN A NUTSHELL 117

- CHAPTER 14: BE REALISTIC 122
- CHAPTER 15: TREATMENT OPTIONS 126
- CHAPTER 16: INTRODUCTION: WHAT IS ADHD? 133
- CHAPTER 17: UNDERSTANDING ADHD'S IMPACT 141
- CHAPTER 18: ATTENTION: DEFICIT OR SURPLUS? 146
- CHAPTER 19: TREATMENT THROUGH LIFESTYLE CHANGES AND HABITS 151
- CHAPTER 20: HELPING CHILDREN WITH ADHD 163
- CHAPTER 21: THE "FEW FOODS" DIET 167
- CHAPTER 22: HOW I INFLUENCE MY CHILD'S BEHAVIOR 171
- CONCLUSION 181

Introduction

First let me congratulate you! Congratulations on your decision to change your life for the better in spite of the difficulties, you may be struggling with. My story also started with me beginning to read. Because I had had enough! Enough of always making excuses for my forgetfulness. Enough of always being afraid of losing my job. Enough of always having to lie about my condition.
Sometimes when my wife asks me to take out the garbage, I find myself with a watering can in my hand, watering chili plants. The garbage bag is left in the utility room because here I found the empty coke bottle I had long promised her that I would throw out. I was moving the coke bottle to the couch when I saw my chili plants were drooping. They needed

watering urgently before they completely dried out ...

Half an hour after I was asked to take out the garbage, I had managed to rearrange my chaos and once again used up a good part of my wife's (almost) limitless patience.

Living with ADHD may require large efforts, not only from oneself but also from loved ones. Many relationships deteriorate over time, as it can be exhausting for both parties. The worst thing is that most adults with these problems do not even realize that they are in fact suffering from ADHD. They do not know that they actually could have done something about it.

But do not despair, there is hope! This book will help you gain insight into what it means to have ADHD and how to ease your daily life with a few simple tools and some good habits. I will in this book go through some methods and strategies to train you to better weather a distracting day with ADHD. Techniques that will ease your daily life so much that you will again dare to dream of a life of structure, yes even success.

Chapter 1: What Parents Need To Know

Attention Deficit Hyperactivity Disorder is a state of the brain that makes it hard for children to control their behavior. All children have issues with their behavior every once in a while, however, kids with ADHD have behavior issues that meddle with regular life and are ceaseless. Kids with ADHD can have various types of indications:

Inattention: These children experience difficulty with focusing, are complicated or stare off into space excessively.

Hyperactivity: These children are continually moving, cannot take a seat or talk excessively.

Impulsivity: These children demonstration and talk without considering, interfere with a great deal or demonstrate misguided thinking.

Combination: The above indications can happen in various mixes.

ADHD and learning inabilities are two various types of conditions, they do co-exist and one might hear these called by the restorative term co-morbidities.

ADHD is the most widely recognized conduct disorder in school-aged children. The definite reasons for ADHD are not yet known. Specialists imagine that ADHD is brought on by contrasts in the way messages are sent to the brain. ADHD appears to keep running in families, so it might be acquired.

ADHD is normally analyzed in school-aged children, ages 6-12, since it is difficult to analyze in children less than 6. The symptomatic procedure has numerous methods, and you, your child's school and different care providers will all have to give data about your kid's conduct.

The best treatment for ADHD is generally pharmaceutical, joined with conduct treatment (including coaching parents in behavior therapy) and setting things up for your kid at home and at school to make it simpler to focus. Since ADHD is an interminable (on-going) condition, treatment should likewise be on-going. Normally, you will have a long-term approach that incorporates objectives for your kid. When every one of the parts of the treatment approaches are set up, and everybody (your kid, parents, educators, specialists, care providers, and so forth) cooperates, treatment will be best.

If your kid is finding it hard in school, approach your educational system in composing an assessment of your kid. They are required to give it, at no expense to you. The motivation behind an assessment is to discover why your kid is not doing admirably in school. A group of experts will work with you to assess your kid. If they do not discover an issue, you can approach the educational system to pay for an assessment. You can likewise have your kid assessed again privately and pay for it yourself. However, check with your school first to ensure they will acknowledge the privately tested results. By law, the educational system must consider the consequences of the second assessment when choosing if your kid can get special services.

In the event that testing demonstrates your kid to have ADHD, the educational system may begin your kid in a specialized curriculum program.

Custom curriculum signifies instructive programming planned particularly for the person. It can truly help your kid improve in school. If your school-aged kid fits the bill for a specialized curriculum, they will have an Individualized Education Plan (IEP) composed only for them.

Medicines and children are among the news lately. A few people think that drugs are endorsed excessively. Others see it working and think it is an incredible thought. Whatever your emotions, make sure you know the fundamental certainties about ADHD meds. Stimulant meds like Ritalin, Dexedrine and Adderall have been utilized for quite a while and have a decent reputation.

There are additionally different sorts of solution that your kid's specialist may attempt if the stimulants do not work. Sometimes, your kid's specialist may need to attempt a couple of various drugs at different dosages to identify the one that works best for your kid. You could think about the brain as a black box that we cannot see inside. The specialist does not know how a solution will influence the mind until he or she tries it. The vast majority of children enhance stimulant prescription.

If your kid's specialist recommends a medication for your kid, ensure you get some information about the advantages and dangers of taking the medication. In the event that your kid is simply beginning prescription, you can utilize a sheet to monitor how they are doing and impart it to your kid's specialist at your next office visit.

You may feel edgy for a silver bullet that will cure your kid's issue. A portion of the alternative medicines may sound sensible and may even be created by specialists or authorities.

However, in the event that they are not experimentally demonstrated, you risk investing energy, money and trust on false guarantees. Then again, you and your kid's specialist may choose it is justified, despite all the trouble to attempt an alternative medicine treatment.

A few medicines that the National Institute of Mental Health and the American Academy of Pediatrics cautions have not been demonstrated to work in exploratory studies are:

Restricted diets

Allergy medications

Medications for motion sickness to treat inner ear issues

Mega-vitamin and mineral supplements

Special hued glasses

EEG biofeedback

Some alternative medications, for example, vitamins and exceptional supplements, may really be risky to your kid. Use prudence and chat with your kid's specialist if you are thinking about alternative and supplemental medicines. Your kid's specialist needs to know all medicines being utilized, as some may interfere with recommended medications.

Biofeedback could be a valuable treatment for ADHD. Biofeedback has the additional advantage of getting children effectively involved in building up their own adapting methodologies. However, biofeedback treatments can be costly, particularly if your insurance does not cover it.

Tips for parents of children with ADHD

Try to concentrate on your kid's great qualities. Catch your kid doing well no less than three times each day and let them know you took note. Work up to more than three times each day.

When you catch your kid, basically depict to them the conduct you saw that you would like to see more frequently.

Tell your child what you need them to do, rather than what you do not need them to do.

Your kid with ADHD will require feedback from you. Give prompt, useful input regularly for the duration of the day. Once again, keep it brief, particular and unmistakable.

Kids with ADHD experience difficulty eating admirably in view of their medications and inconvenience sitting still. Ensure your youngster gets adequate meals and healthy snacks.

Vigorous activity is additionally extremely accommodating for your kid, yet ensures they stay safe. Kids with ADHD should be observed more intently than different children their age since they can be dynamic and incautious. There are sure things you ought to do to keep them safe, similar to ensure they wear a helmet when biking or roller-blading.

Kids with ADHD frequently experience difficulty sleeping. Realize what to do when your kid has issues with sleep.

Help your kid develop great social and relational abilities, which will help them to form satisfying fellowships with different children.

Make beyond any doubt your kid's different care providers are likewise acquainted with day by day schedules and behavioral objectives. This will guarantee that your kid gets consistency for the duration of the day.

Behavior related tips:

Do not attempt to change number of behaviors at one go. Target one to three behaviors at a time to deal with.

Talk about the behavioral objectives with your kid.

You will presumably need to concentrate intently on target behavior for tracking and feedback for 60 minutes a day or for limited period of time on a general schedule. Doing this throughout the day is excessively overwhelming for both you and your kid.

Reward your kid with benefits and extraordinary activities like an outing to the recreation center or a family excursion for effectively meeting behavioral objectives.

Keep a limited set of rules and execute them reliably.

Offer alternate decisions, however, keep them basic.

Tips to set up the house:

Keep a consistent routine and give heaps of structure, so your kid comprehends what is in store.

Post records and updates for the schedules in key spots around the house. For instance, you may keep a rundown of things to convey to school by the front entryway or in your kid's knapsack.

Keep your home sorted out. Store things as close as could be allowed to where they are utilized, and have a spot for everything and everything in its place.

Tips to get child's attention:

No shouting directions from the other room while you are accomplishing something else. You definitely realize that does not work in any case.

To stand out enough to be noticed, get down on the floor before the kid, and put your hands on the shoulders. When you kid look at you, let you kid know what you have to say.

When you give directions, give them each one in turn. Separate difficult tasks into a few smaller tasks.

Repeat your directions with good eye contact. Hope to need to rehash yourself again and again.

Try composing a list of items for different tasks and separate challenging tasks into do-able pieces.

Tips to adapt to the difficulties of bringing up a kid with ADHD:

Teachers will change every year, except parents are dependably there. That is the reason you are your kid's ideal and most essential educator.

Plan for one-on-one time with your kid every day. Indeed, even 10-15 minutes consistently will go far in telling your kid they are extraordinary to you. Take after your kid's lead in the middle of this extraordinary time. This will help both of you feel associated and cherishing toward each other.

Stay quiet and in control of yourself. You cannot constrain your youngster to carry on the way you need them to, yet you are in complete control of your own conduct.

Act the way you need your kid to act. Be a decent good example.

Get support. There is a great deal of different parents out there experiencing the same thing as you, and you can help each other with thoughts and just by tuning in.

Tips to help kid improve in school:

Keep in close touch with your kid's teacher and cooperate to make things as steady as could be expected under the circumstances at school and at home. Get involved and help the teacher as much as could reasonably be expected.

In some cases your kid's instructors will be exceptionally proficient and accommodating, and sometimes they would not. However, it helps a lot if you learn as much as you can about ADHD, and offer with your kid's teacher on what works best for your kid. You might need to share the tips for teachers in the following segment with your kid's teacher.

Tips for teachers to help kids with ADHD:

An educator who comprehends ADHD and how to function with children with ADHD will have a major effect in your kid's school experience. Educators need to see how to utilize a project of scholastic direction, behavioral mediations and classroom lodging to help kids with ADHD. You may need to help your kid's educator take in more about how to function best with your kid at school. Some essential tips for changing the classroom include:

Seating the youngster close to the educator
Repeating guidelines
Not putting time limits on test and tests
Helping the youngster arrange
Boosting the youngster's self-regard
Having steady outcomes for inadmissible conduct.

Educators may acknowledge realizing that numerous assets exist that can help them learn new methodologies to show kids with ADHD.

Chapter 2: Adhd, Its Signs, Symptoms And Treatment

What is ADHD?

ADHD (Attention deficit hyperactivity Disorder) is a mental disorder that affects children and teens. Children with this disorder have a disruptive behaviour and are unable to control their reactions and impulses. Such kids are usually hyperactive and can't focus well. They have difficulty in paying attention and generally act without thinking.

ADHD is known to affect children and teenagers. This condition can continue very much into the adulthood. Adults with ADHD are not organized and can't manage their time, goals and relationships well.

ADHD does not have a single cause, but researches found that it can be caused by hereditary issues and chemical imbalances in the brain. A brain injury or disorder could be another cause.

Though it can't be cured or prevented, but an early analysis can help the child or adult diagnosed with ADHD to manage his lifestyle well.

SIGNS and SYMPTOMS

How would you know if your child or a child you know is having ADHD? There are some tell-tale signs that you should look out for. These signs and symptoms will help you to recognize ADHD.

The signs and symptoms of ADHD in children are as follows:

1. **Hyperactive** – The child is fidgety and has a problem to remain seated for a long duration. He is always on the move and shows his restlessness behaviour by trying to run or climb on various things. The child squirms, talks a lot and plays quite noisily.

2. **Inattention** – The child is forgetful and has problems focusing on daily activities. He doesn't listen, remains distracted and fails to pay attention on things. The child will often make careless mistakes and leave his tasks incomplete.

3. **Impulsive** – The child is quite impulsive and tends to interrupt other people when they are speaking. He has issues with waiting for his own turn.

Other conditions linked to ADHD

ADHD is known to coexist with other medical conditions. About two-thirds of kids diagnosed with ADHD are also known to suffer from other medical disorders. Most of the children who are diagnosed with ADHD are also known to have at least one of the following conditions:

Learning disabilities: About 40-50% of kids diagnosed with ADHD also have a learning disorder. The kids could have a difficulty in understanding words and sounds. As the kids grow, they could experience difficulty in writing, reading and expressing themselves.

Oppositional defiant disorder: Research has proved as about 30-40% of kids with ADHD also show symptoms of oppositional defiant disorder. A child with oppositional defiant disorder will have a problem with authority and would often disregard authoritative figures.

Autism: Many studies have known to prove that about half of the children with ASD (Autism Spectrum Disorders) have ADHD. There is a strong connection between autism and ADHD. Children battling with autism struggle to interact and communicate well. It impairs the social, emotional, physical and cognitive health of the child.

Tourette disorder: A few kids with ADHD could also have the Tourette disorder. The child with Tourette disorder is unable to control certain sounds and movements. The child could make repetitive sounds and movements, such as blinking of eyes.

Conduct disorder: Conduct disorder is a very serious disorder because children known to have Conduct disorder tend to lie and steal. This can hamper their social life. It can be very difficult for the parents and teachers to manage such kids. About

40-50% of kids battling with the condition of ADHD also have Conduct disorder.

Speech and language disorders: ADHD has a very strong connection with speech and language disorders. ADHD affects the ability of a child to concentrate and pay attention. This in turn affects his speech and language. Most kids with ADHD are known to suffer from speech and language disorders. For example, the kids diagnosed with ADHD can experience the problem of speech delay.

Depression: It is known that about 25% of kids with ADHD also suffer from depression. It is important that the warning signs of depression are recognized and treated to help the kids deal with ADHD.

Bipolarity: A few kids with ADHD also develop bipolar disorder, where they experience extreme mood swings. Such kids will experience alternate phases of extreme happiness and depression.

As the child develops into an adult, the symptoms can also undergo some changes and can get a little complicated. The signs and symptoms in adults are:

The person suffers from low self-esteem, forgetfulness, anxiety and impulsiveness.

He cannot control his anger, gets irritated and frustrated easily.

He tends to have problems while concentrating on things and also has issues at his work place.

The person can suffer from serious depression and can even be a victim to substance abuse.

The person can have problems in his personal relationships. Such people are also known to suffer from drastic mood swings.

He procrastinate his work and is often restless and unorganized.

Treatment

Though ADHD can't be cured, it can be managed well. It is important to have personalized sessions and follow ups with the doctor. The doctor will effectively use a combination of behavioural therapy and medicines to manage ADHD. The family should learn to accept the child, his condition as well as help him to control his reactions and behaviour.

Medications:

The medicines that can be used in the treatment of ADHD fall under the following categories:

1) **Stimulants** – Stimulants have been used in ADHD treatment for more than 50 years. They can help to control impulsiveness and hyperactivity. Stimulants include medicines such as Dexmethylphenidate and Methylphenidate. Stimulants are known to have a few side effects, such as insomnia, reduced appetite and stomach ache. Their effect can last from a minimum of 4 hours to a maximum of up to 12 hours.

2) **Non stimulants** – They can be prescribed for those above the age of 6 years. They are known to have fewer side

effects when compared with stimulants, and their effect can last up to a maximum of 24 hours. A combination of stimulants and non-stimulants can be used for effective management of ADHD. Non-stimulants include medicines such as Atomoxetine and Clonidine.

3) **Antidepressants** – Antidepressants can also be used, but their effects and side effects should be thoroughly discussed with the doctor first before using them, as antidepressants can have some major side effects on children.

Different children react differently to different medicines. The doctor might prescribe different doses of various medicines to check what works best for the child.

Behavioural therapy:

Medications are generally taken with a combination of behavioural therapy. This therapy is used to change the patterns of the child's behaviour by:

Encouraging the child to discipline himself and to follow a routine

Setting rewards for certain behaviour, so as to abstain the child from negative behaviour

Rearranging the child's environment according to his needs, be it school or home

Giving brief and clear instructions to children

Counselling can go a long way in improving the child's self confidence

Teaching the child the difference between good behaviour and bad behaviour

Chiropractic Care

Chiropractic care follows a holistic approach towards treatment. Chiropractic neurologists treat their patients without any medications. They perform brain function tests on the patient to identify the brain's hypo functioning part. This helps them to diagnose which environmental stimuli can affect the brain.

Chiropractic care can be very useful with patients with ADHD, especially those with sensory issues. Doctors spend a lot of time with the patients to understand the various types of factors interfering with the body's natural healing mechanism. An imbalance of the muscle tone can cause nerve irritability, which can lead to agitation and other issues with the nervous system. Every ADHD patient is unique, so it is important to identify the patient's individual symptoms. The physical examination of the child includes checking for divergences, disorganizations and tactility and auditory issues. A child with reading issues has a communication gap between the two sides of the body, whereas a child with vision problems has a divergence issue.

With the physical examination, it is important to look for emotional and chemical issues that affect the child. Stool analysis and blood chemistry of the child is used to check sensitivities related to food.

The emotional issue that the patient is going through should also be addressed with care.

Art therapy can also be used to treat the children. The child can be asked to draw pictures on a sheet of paper, in order to express how he feels. This can help the child to let out his emotions and channelize them in a creative direction.

A few ADHD children can have issues with the texture of some food items. The chiropractic adjustments in such children can help to reduce the issue of their sensitivity. This reduction in sensitivity will reduce the distractions and further improve the attention span of the child. The child will be less irritated, and thus can focus in a better way.

Chapter 3: What Is Adhd?

Understanding ADHD is, part of the battle already won as it pertains to ensuring that your kid can live a productive and full life even if they have been identified as having this very common childhood illness. So what exactly is Attention Deficit/Hyperactivity Disorder (ADHD) anyway and what are the symptoms that signal your kid may have ADHD?

If you type the phrase: "what is ADHD" into an internet search engine, you'll be certain to get plenty of results. ADHD or Attention Deficit/Hyperactivity Disorder is a very common ailment that is understood to continue throughout the kid's adolescent years and on into their adult years at the same time as it pertains to childhood disorders. Badly disciplined, boisterous, etc., when left untreated, the symptoms associated with the illness can make life quite hard for the kid who's regularly berated for being lazy, unwilling to work; as adults the symptoms can make holding onto a job difficult and there is difficulty in keeping relationships that are healthy too. The symptoms of Attention Deficit/Hyperactivity Disorder truly reflect ordinary behavior in a lot of manners which makes identification a difficulty. It is because of this that comprehensive and appropriate appraisals by professionals that are skilled, are crucial to ascertain whether a child has ADHD or not. It is important that you know that there is no single test that will determine if your child has ADHD.

So what is ADHD?

To understand what ADHD is, one has to first become acquainted with the symptoms of this disorder. The symptoms can be divided into three sub-categories:

1. Mainly Hyperactive/Impulsive
2. Mostly Inattentive
3. Combined Hyperactive/Impulsive and Inattentive

Most children clinically determined to have ADHD fall into the third category. Symptoms include:

1. Fidgeting
2. Difficulty concentrating for any length of time thereby unable to complete a task.
3. Issue focusing on action or a job for long periods of time.
4. Losing interest in a job or activity.
5. Losing tools and items necessary to complete a job or activity.
6. Propensity to jump and run around even at inopportune times.
7. Constantly on the run.
8. Unruly behavior such as shouting out answers before the question is completely asked.
9. Trouble sleeping.

Now you know more about ADHD, the treatment choices which are available will be revolved around by the next question probably to be asked. Normally the mental health professional will want to put the child on one or more drugs to combat the symptoms of the illness. It is essential to understand that there's no treatment for this ailment and the only recourse will be to manage the symptoms so that the kid is therefore able to perform better academically and to focus and concentrate better. While the medications prescribed can indeed be helpful in treating the disorder and handling the symptoms, and many children benefit from taking them, there are also issues surrounding their safety given the fact that many of them can be highly addictive and dangerous with rather unpleasant side effects. Nevertheless, when a kid is on treatment, whether this is achieved via medication or through treatments and alternate remedies, it is possible for the child to lead a normal and healthy life. Scientists and researchers today are continuously investigating and researching the illness so as to develop more effective treatments and even interventions.

Many individuals are turning to alternative ways of combating and reducing the symptoms of ADHD and these are proving to be highly effective along with being far safer, although it is essential to talk to your child's doctor before any treatment is undertaken. This is especially true if the child has already been on an ADHD drug. It truly is crucial if, this really is your choice the child be weaned off the drug slowly. Although science has yet to corroborate it, many people have found that altering the kid's diet can have great advantages on minimizing the symptoms of the disorder and when combined with other remedies, such as relaxation techniques, exercise, supplements, etc., can have quite valuable and long lasting effects.

ADHD Subtypes

ADHD has primarily three (3) subtypes.

Predominantly hyperactive-impulsive

With this subtype, most of the symptoms - six or more - are classified under the hyperactivity-impulsivity categories.

Additionally, although symptoms of attention may still be present, they are usually less than six (6).

Predominantly inattentive

The majority of symptoms in this subtype (six or more) are in the inattention category and fewer than six symptoms of hyperactivity-impulsivity are present, although hyperactivity-impulsivity may still be present to some degree.

Children with this subtype are less likely to act out or have difficulties getting along with other children. They may sit quietly, although not paying attention to what they are doing. Therefore, the child may be overlooked, and parents and teachers may not notice that he or she has ADHD.

Combined hyperactive-impulsive and inattentive

Six or more symptoms of inattention and six or more symptoms of hyperactivity-impulsivity are present.

REAL AND ROMOURED CAUSES

The jury is still out in the scientific community as to the exact causes of ADHD, although many studies suggest that genes play a large role. Like many other illnesses, ADHD most likely results from more than a single factor. Genetics aside, researchers are looking at possible environmental factors, and are studying how brain injuries, nutrition, and the social environment might contribute to ADHD.

Was It From Mum And Dad?

Results from several international studies of twins show that ADHD often runs in families, so, yes, it could be from mum or day!

Researchers are looking at several genes that seem to predispose a person to developing this disorder. By knowing and isolating the genes involved, it is anticipated that scientist in the not too distant future could develop methods of preventing the onset of ADHD symptoms. This knowledge could also lead to better treatments.

Children with ADHD who carry a particular version of a certain gene have thinner brain tissue in the areas of the brain associated with attention. This NIMH research showed that the difference was not permanent, however, and as children with this gene grew up, the brain developed to a normal level of thickness. Their ADHD symptoms also improved.

What's Environmental factors Got To Do With ADHD?

Studies suggest a potential link between cigarette smoking and alcohol use during pregnancy and ADHD in children. In ADHDition, preschoolers who are exposed to high levels of lead, which can sometimes be found in plumbing fixtures or paint in old buildings, may have a higher risk of developing ADHD.

Could It Be The Brain injuries?

Children who have suffered a brain injury may show some behaviors similar to those of ADHD. However, only a small percentage of children with ADHD have suffered a traumatic brain injury.

Refined Sugar?

The idea that refined sugar causes ADHD or makes symptoms worse is popular, but more research discounts this theory than supports it. In one study, researchers gave children foods containing either sugar or a sugar substitute every other day. The children who received sugar showed no different behavior or learning capabilities than those who received the sugar substitute. Another study in which children were given higher than average amounts of sugar or sugar substitutes showed similar results.

In another study, children who were considered sugar-sensitive by their mothers were given the sugar substitute aspartame, also known as Nutrasweet. Although all the children got aspartame, half their mothers were told their children were given sugar, and the other half were told their children were given aspartame.

The mothers who thought their children had gotten sugar rated them as more hyperactive than the other children and were more critical of their behavior, compared to mothers who thought their children received aspartame.

Food Additives

Recent British research indicates a possible link between consumption of certain food additives like artificial colors or preservatives, and an increase in activity. Research is under way to confirm the findings and to learn more about how food additives may affect hyperactivity.

TRUE SIGNS & SYMPTOMS

Inattention, hyperactivity, and impulsivity are the key behaviors of ADHD. Although it is to be expected that children be inattentive, hyperactive, or impulsive, for children with ADHD, these behaviors are more pronounced and occur more often.

To be diagnosed with the disorder, a child must have symptoms for 6 or more months and to a degree that is greater than other children of the same age.

Children who have symptoms of inattention may:

Be easily distracted, miss details, forget things, and frequently switch from one activity to another

Have difficulty focusing on one thing

Become bored with a task after only a few minutes, unless they are doing something enjoyable

Have difficulty focusing attention on organizing and completing a task or learning something new

Have trouble completing or turning in homework assignments, often losing things (e.g., pencils, toys, assignments) needed to complete tasks or activities

Not seem to listen when spoken to

Daydream, become easily confused, and move slowly

Have difficulty processing information as quickly and accurately as others

Struggle to follow instructions.

Children who have symptoms of hyperactivity may:
Fidget and squirm in their seats
Talk nonstop
Dash around, touching or playing with anything and everything in sight
Have trouble sitting still during dinner, school, and story time
Be constantly in motion
Have difficulty doing quiet tasks or activities.
Children who have symptoms of impulsivity may:
Be very impatient
Blurt out inappropriate comments, show their emotions without restraint, and act without regard for consequences
Have difficulty waiting for things they want or waiting their turns in games
Often interrupt conversations or other people's activities.
ADHD Can Be Mistaken for Other Problems

Parents and teachers can miss the fact that children with symptoms of inattention have the disorder because they are often quiet and less likely to act out. They may sit quietly, seeming to work, but they are often not paying attention to what they are doing. They may get along well with other children, compared with those with the other subtypes, who tend to have social problems. But children with the inattentive kind of ADHD are not the only ones whose disorders can be missed. For example, adults may think that children with the hyperactive and impulsive subtypes just have emotional or disciplinary problems.

Chapter 4: Science And Real Life

ADD (Attention Deficit Disorder) and ADHD (Attention Deficit Hyperactivity Disorder) are controversial issues and will probably remain so for decades to come. The main reason is a discrepancy between real-life situations and problems for people that ADHD symptoms, and the statistically general and over simplified models for a complex condition.

The symptoms of ADHD are defined in the DSM-IV (Diagnostic and Statistical Manual of Mental Disorders fourth edition) in a categorical manner. This is useful for research, but vary in real life ADHD symptoms in a three dimensional way.

The signs and symptoms vary in size for each individual:

· ADHD symptoms vary in the combination of symptoms he or she has.
· ADHD symptoms vary in the severity of each of these symptoms.
· ADHD symptoms vary in what develops the cause of the symptoms in the first place.
· ADHD symptoms vary in the personal views of the evaluation of attention deficit and hyperactive behavior.

- ADHD symptoms vary in experiential experience of the person's attention deficit symptoms and / or hyperactivity.

Statistics are useful in seeing the overall picture, but the statistics are not always relevant when applied to an individual. There is also confusion caused by the mixing of various medical, physiological and psychological disorders in the same category as the true ADHD personality.

True ADHD people are cognitively attention deficit hyper-intuitive but can focus, which is a talent and one of their many strengths. Unfortunately, they are not able to choose what condition they are in, or will power by choice, but the state they are in at any time depends on situations. Therefore ADHD behavior and causes situational problems.

Scientific research focuses on the problems. How do they get by watching the funding for their research on the bright side? But we who have ADHD need to focus on solutions. There are strengths and talents embedded in the ADHD personality. For this reason we find a better self-understanding.

Understanding of ourselves as individuals, to accept that we are different and channeling our energy, enthusiasm and creativity in our strengths while developing coping strategies for our weaknesses, are the keys to living successful and fulfilled lives with ADHD.

There is a solution for you or your child with ADHD. But there is no perfect universal treatment or cure for the problems associated with ADD and ADHD because there are so many factors that can sometimes lead to a complicated or confusing diagnosis. Each of us that has attention deficit disorder, needs to find the right combination of natural ADHD treatments that fits each of us as an individual.

Because there are so many causes of ADHD behaviors and symptoms, more than one hundred, we need to know first if there is a medical or psychological cause of the symptoms of ADHD. If the problem is, for example, the thyroid gland, which may result in either inattention or hyperactivity, then that must be dealt with, not the attention deficit symptoms.

There are natural treatments and cures for ADHD problems. Specially formulated supplements, behavioral strategies and coping strategies are the basis of these courses. Because ADHD signs are situational, lifestyle changes, where we live, we spend the most time with and career, taking the strengths of the ADHD personality into account, can make huge differences in personal satisfaction.

Given that we have more time to spend in our workshop or company than any other activity, an ADHD personality should choose a career in which he / she can put their heart and soul into. A work that is stimulating with minimal tasks that challenge struggling attention deficit personality, gives energy and leads to creativity.

This may sound radical. But in the long term these decisions, using our individual combination of ADHD symptoms as clues to go in that direction, will lead to a life where the gifts and strengths of our attention deficit hyper-focused character can be a joy.

Chapter 5: The Introduction Of Benzedrine

The U.S. Food and Drug Administration (FDA) approved Benzedrine as a medicine in 1936. Dr. Charles Bradley stumbled across some unexpected side effects of this medicine the next year. Young patients' behavior and performance in school improved when he gave it to them.

However, Bradley's contemporaries largely ignored his findings. Doctors and researchers began to recognize the benefit of what Bradley had discovered many years later.

No recognition

The APA issued the first "Diagnostic and Statistical Manual of Mental Disorders" (DSM) in 1952. This manual listed all of the recognized mental disorders. It also included known causes, risk factors, and treatments for each condition. Doctors still use an updated version today.

The APA did not recognize ADHD in the first edition. A second DSM was published in 1968. This edition included hyperkinetic impulse disorder for the first time.

The introduction of Ritalin

The FDA approved the psychostimulant Ritalin (methylphenidate) in 1955. It became more popular as an ADHD treatment as the disorder became better understood and diagnoses increased. The medicine is still used to treat ADHD today.

A changing definition

The APA released a third edition of the DSM (DSM-III) in 1980. They changed the name of the disorder from hyperkinetic impulse disorder to attention deficit disorder (ADD). Scientists believed hyperactivity was not a common symptom of the disorder. This listing created two subtypes of ADD: ADD with hyperactivity, and ADD without hyperactivity.

Finally, a name that fits

The APA released a revised version of the DSM-III in 1987. They removed the hyperactivity distinction and changed the name to attention deficit hyperactivity disorder (ADHD). The APA combined the three symptoms (inattentiveness, impulsivity, and hyperactivity) into a single type and did not identify subtypes of the disorder.

The APA released the fourth edition of the DSMin 2000. The fourth edition established the three subtypes of ADHD used by healthcare professionals today:

combined type ADHD

predominantly inattentive type ADHD

predominantly hyperactive-impulsive type ADHD

A climb in diagnoses

ADHD cases began to climb significantly in the 1990s. There may be a few factors behind the rise in diagnoses:

doctors were able to diagnose ADHD more efficiently

more parents were aware of ADHD and are reporting their children's symptoms more children were actually developing ADHD

More and more medications to treat the disorder became available as the number of ADHD cases rose. The medications also became more effective at treating ADHD. Many have long-acting benefits for patients who need relief from symptoms for longer periods.

Where we are today

Scientists are trying to identify the causes of ADHD as well as possible treatments. Research points to a very strong genetic link. Children who have parents or siblings with the disorder are more likely to have it.

It's not currently clear what role environmental factors play in determining who develops ADHD. Researchers are dedicated to finding the underlying cause of the disorder. They're aiming to make treatments more effective and to help find cures.

Attention-deficit/hyperactivity disorder (ADHD) is a chronic condition that affects millions of children and often continues into adulthood. ADHD includes a combination of persistent problems, such as difficulty sustaining attention, hyperactivity and impulsive behavior.

Children with ADHD may also struggle with low self-esteem, troubled relationships and poor performance in school. Symptoms sometimes lessen with age. However, some people never completely outgrow their ADHD symptoms. But they can learn strategies to be successful.

While treatment won't cure ADHD, it can help a great deal with symptoms. Treatment typically involves medications and behavioral interventions. Early diagnosis and treatment can make a big difference in outcome.

Symptoms

The primary features of ADHD include inattention and hyperactive-impulsive behavior. ADHD symptoms start before age 12, and in some children, they're noticeable as early as 3 years of age. ADHD symptoms can be mild, moderate or severe, and they may continue into adulthood.

ADHD occurs more often in males than in females, and behaviors can be different in boys and girls. For example, boys may be more hyperactive and girls may tend to be quietly inattentive. There are three subtypes of ADHD:

Predominantly inattentive. The majority of symptoms fall under inattention.

Predominantly hyperactive/impulsive. The majority of symptoms are hyperactive and impulsive.

Combined. This is a mix of inattentive symptoms and hyperactive/impulsive symptoms.

Inattention

A child who shows a pattern of inattention may often:

Fail to pay close attention to details or make careless mistakes in schoolwork

Have trouble staying focused in tasks or play

Appear not to listen, even when spoken to directly

Have difficulty following through on instructions and fail to finish schoolwork or chores

Have trouble organizing tasks and activities

Avoid or dislike tasks that require focused mental effort, such as homework

Lose items needed for tasks or activities, for example, toys, school assignments, pencils

Be easily distracted

Forget to do some daily activities, such as forgetting to do chores

Hyperactivity and impulsivity

A child who shows a pattern of hyperactive and impulsive symptoms may often:

Fidget with or tap his or her hands or feet, or squirm in the seat

Have difficulty staying seated in the classroom or in other situations
Be on the go, in constant motion
Run around or climb in situations when it's not appropriate
Have trouble playing or doing an activity quietly
Talk too much
Blurt out answers, interrupting the questioner
Have difficulty waiting for his or her turn
Interrupt or intrude on others' conversations, games or activities

Typical developmental behavior vs. ADHD

Most healthy children are inattentive, hyperactive or impulsive at one time or another. It's typical for preschoolers to have short attention spans and be unable to stick with one activity for long. Even in older children and teenagers, attention span often depends on the level of interest.

The same is true of hyperactivity. Young children are naturally energetic they often are still full of energy long after they've worn their parents out. In addition, some children just naturally have a higher activity level than others do.

Children should never be classified as having ADHD just because they're different from their friends or siblings. Children who have problems in school but get along well at home or with friends are likely struggling with something other than ADHD. The same is true of children who are hyperactive or inattentive at home, but whose schoolwork and friendships remain unaffected.

When to see a doctor

If you're concerned that your child shows signs of ADHD, see your pediatrician or family doctor. Your doctor may refer you to a specialist, such as a developmental-behavioral pediatrician, psychologist, psychiatrist or pediatric neurologist, but it's important to have a medical evaluation first to check for other possible causes of your child's difficulties.

Chapter 6: Add: How Is It Different From Adhd?

Attention Deficit Disorder or ADD is a very complicated, and time and again misinterpreted, disorder. Its beginning is physiological, but it can have a multitude of consequences that come alongside with it. That apart, what is the differentiation between ADHD and ADD? ADHD is the abbreviated form of Attention Deficit Hyperactive Disorder, its major indications being noticeable hyperactivity and impulsivity. These are the indications that are noticeable to the purposeful onlooker. ADD stands for Attention Deficit Disorder with the major indications being lack of concentration. Now a lot of other things can come alongside with both of these subtypes of ADHD, but those are the distinctive characteristics of both.

For several years, the usual picture of Attention Deficit Disorder has been the little boy that is bouncing off the walls and making his teachers and parents go mad. ADHD is beyond a doubt the more identifiable of the two subtypes since it is so much more noticeable than ADD. Since hyperactivity causes a lot more disruption and problems for classrooms, it gets the most notice and will be picked up on a lot quicker. Unluckily, even if ADD is less visible, the consequences of the disorder can just as negative.

With negligent attention deficit disorder, or ADD, the person enduring it will give the impression of being spacey and disordered. More often, victims with this type will be gazing out of the window during classes and will seem as if they are never somewhat there. It is much more tricky to make a diagnosis and a lot of people with this form of ADD go years without even knowing they have it. But the consequences of the drifting mind can be just as disparaging.

For a long time, it was considered that only boys suffered from ADHD. However, this figment has been busted of late. It is now acknowledged that both girls and boys can suffer from attention deficit disorder, and many do not get out of it in middle age. One disparity that has been noticed is that girls are inclined to have the inattentive version of ADD, and many times it is wrongly diagnosed as depression. Since inattentive ADD does not create noticeable troubles and disruptions to the nearby surroundings, a lot of them endure in silence for years before they discover the real reason of their plight.

With both ADHD and ADD, making a diagnosis early on is very essential. Even though troubles with schools are the most apparent indications, some victims do not have major problems with

Understanding And Treating ADHD

getting school work completed. Keep track of your children, not just academically, but generally and psychologically as well. Do they have problem with other children?

Does it appear as if they have difficulty putting in order or are extremely disordered? Do they have difficulty sitting motionless for a period of time? Are they extremely silent or extremely chatty? Now any of these indications do not in particular denote ADD or ADHD, but they do point to asking for outside help from a therapist or a counselor.

Your child's psychological well being is just as vital as their physical well being and how they do in school. Confirm it out if you sense like something is off. If left for years not diagnosed, ADD can create a lot of other resulting troubles that can take a long time to get rid off and can be arrested.

Understanding And Treating ADHD

ADD: The Types Of Its Manifestation In Kids

Attention Deficit Disorder can take several forms in children. It is not difficult to track the child with ADD who is very chaotic. Boys generally come into this category.

But then there are some types of ADD which go undiagnosed because their effects in children are less outwardly evident. This happens mainly in case of girls.

There are many girls who are called "tomboys". They frequently exhibit some of the important features off ADD, like being more involved in physical activities, but not as reckless as the boys themselves. As a result teachers and parents jump to the conclusion that the child has no interest in academics and is basically not organized, but the possibility of ADD is seldom considered.

Besides the "tomboy" types, the "chatty" girls could also be suffering from ADD, but remaining undiagnosed. This is a fusion of over-activity and inattentiveness, and is usually touted as socially extrovert. These girls are extremely talkative than being physically active and cannot stop talking even if they are strictly warned. They also cannot tell stories comprehensively and will stray from their thoughts because of ADD.

Those whom we call as "daydreamers" could also be suffering from ADD. They do not draw any attention to themselves and are very quite in nature. However, their too much being into themselves and not giving any attention to the class is another form of ADD, contrary to the "chatty" girls. They may show anxiety and depression when given school projects, but cannot finish the projects because of their lack of staying power. This generally goes undiagnosed because the child is thought to be lazy and, parents and teachers fail to identify the disorder in time.

What is fascinating is that many girls with ADD have quite a high rate of IQ and could be called "gifted". When a child has a high IQ there are no problems in school work, but their lack loopholes get reflected as they mature into adults. Keep in mind that ADD is not a learning disorder, and patients do not inevitably are poor performers in school. Till high school they can be quite well off, but with mounting pressure and assignments symptoms may become more and more evident.

Understanding And Treating ADHD

When undiagnosed, Attention Deficit Disorder may cause a lot of harm to an individual. Children will be called unorganized, lacking intelligence and lazy, when in truth, they might be silent sufferers of ADD. They will have very low esteem of themselves, and believe themselves to be quitters or stupid because of their problems. It is crucial that the problem is identifies and treated before it becomes too late and any long-term damage is done.

Understanding And Treating ADHD

Attention Deficit Disorder: Getting Your Facts Right

With all that is written about ADHD, most of us tend to think of a bad little lad running about ruining whatever comes his way. So we often believe that we can spot the child with ADD while we are out. Well the naughty little boy is there fine, but did we ever spare a thought about the little girl who sits quiet and withdrawn with her mother, one who is overtly polite, terribly afraid to speak out and draws a blank when spoken to? In all probabilities, everyone would fail to guess that she might be suffering from ADD or the Attention Deficit Disorder.

Difficult as they are, ADD and ADHD have some obvious symptoms too. The affected person suffers from distraction, easy forgetfulness and low self-esteem, faces problem in following fast conversations and gets highly disordered with tasks. ADD and ADHD both can retard mental growth in this that the affected child has to struggle with school work and assignment deadlines, failing to finish things on time. These disorders also rob the child off his/her ability to manage the belongings and to keep track of time.

ADD Symptoms:

- Lacks vigor, suffers from sloth
- Values others more, respecting their individual limits
- Often unassertive or under-assertive
- Too much obedience
- Excessive humbleness and modesty
- Overtly polite and shy
- Avoiding crowd, preferring to stay alone and socially withdrawn
- Not able to open up easily and befriend, although they make a few bonds

Since it is assumed that girls are generally shy, people often overlook the ADD symptoms in them and they are left untreated. Their outward calm, quiet and politeness are usually to cover up the inner disturbance. ADD affected girls are emotional and highly sensitive to criticism; but the feelings invoked thus, after being criticized, remain untold. They just carry on with life, struggling silently. Interestingly enough, their ADHD counterparts move forward with absolutely no sign of stress or fatigue and seem totally unaffected by all deterrents in the walk of life. Girls

Understanding And Treating ADHD

suffering from ADD cannot withstand stress and usually draw back more into a shell with a belief that they are good-for-nothing and can never do anything right.

Helping a person with ADD
All ADD affected girls are predominantly emotional, irrespective of their nature— be it shy, social, introvert, hyperactive or super-impulsive. This over-sensitivity evidently invites regular upsets which, in turn, give rise to more and more stress. Hence, they should be taught to manage stress through various techniques from an early age. They must also be ascribed a certain revival time to regroup or collect themselves after every damage or emotional upset.

Although it is true that parents always wish the best for their children, they sometimes, unknowingly, impede mental growth in their kids by hurling too much criticism at them or by driving them mad with a series of never-ending do's and don'ts like "You must not be so silly. You got to finish school with high grades", "You need to improve your looks. Try and be as smart as your brother", "You should be a little more assertive. This won't help", "why do you let yourself be taken for granted? Wake up", "Make more friends", "Do not let go off things so easily" so on and so forth. While all these are fine at times, too much of criticism breeds low self-esteem in her—be she shy, outspoken, drawn-back or unruly!

At school, throughout the day, the confidence and self-regard of these girls are constantly shattered and their only respite is at home, where they can rebuild their crushed dignity and revitalize themselves to fight another day. Continuous criticism roots in them the belief that they are worthless. These girls suffering from ADD become extremely impulsive, disorganized and lack focus in everything only to secure poor grades in class. Full of distractions, these girls lack the vigor and energy to develop their personality and skill sets that their peers have. Instead of pointing at their limitations, it is better to compliment them or appreciate when they pick up a skill or show signs of a good ability. Their psyche just needs a positive boost. And it's not hard to make them feel good—an ADD-affected girl can easily get lucky and find interest in some activity. That then becomes the first positive move, the most desired turning point in their lives!

Chapter 7: What The Heck Is Adhd Anyways?

If you or someone close to you suffers from ADHD, then you probably already know that the term itself is a shorter version of "attention deficit/hyperactivity disorder".

As suggested by the name itself, ADHD is a mental condition, or the brain function disorder, which is characterized by impulsive behavior, hyperactivity, and difficulty maintaining attention.

This actually means that the normal functions of the brain are disrupted, resulting in restless behavior, marked by the tendency to forget things, lack of focus, and impulsive, spur-of-the-moment decisions. Even though ADHD is a disorder which primarily affects your behavior and thinking, it consequently affects almost all other areas of your life.

When it comes to some possible causes of ADHD, there seem to be no exact reasons that could be pinpointed as the one responsible for this condition. However, there are some social and biological factors which may put one at risk of developing ADHD.

For instance, some of the studies show that people suffering from this disorder typically have fewer connections between certain parts of the brain. Also, some of the risk factors may cause the development of ADHD while a child is still in the womb.

These factors include smoking during pregnancy, maternal stress, as well as small weight of the baby at birth.

As for social factors, children with low family income and low paternal education belong to that group with a high risk of developing ADHD.

When someone mentions ADHD, one usually associates it with children. However, this is the condition adults suffer from as well. What is in children recognized as hyperactivity may not be observed in adults simply because adults are able to manage their behavior better than children.

On the other hand, adults suffering from ADHD are very often full of some kind of nervous energy, and thus tend to be edgy and restless. Even though in some cases it may go unnoticed, ADHD develops in childhood and the symptoms usually persist into adulthood.

In some rare cases, ADHD may appear in adults who did not have any of the symptoms in their childhood. In such cases, some brain injuries may be the reason for developing ADHD.

The belief is that ADHD is harder to spot in adults since some of the symptoms may easily be misunderstood for some other condition, such as depression, anxiety, or mood swings.

Some other disorders that commonly co-occur with ADHD are autism spectrum disorders, alcoholism and other addictions, conduct disorder, oppositional defiant disorder, and adult antisocial personality.

Even though at first glance ADHD is not like other mental conditions, it really hurts, and it hurts every day. People suffering from ADHD are sometimes thought of as being unintelligent or lazy because of their poor organizational skills, inability to follow directions, lack of concentration, etc.

So, besides some everyday problems and difficulties, people with ADHD have to cope with these prejudices as well.

Summary

ADHD is a mental health condition which affects your behavior and thinking, which may cause you many problems, such as troubles with losing things, keeping appointments, meeting deadlines, getting along with other people, etc.

Chapter 8: Parenting In Public

Nothing can be more anxiety-provoking than a shopping trip with a child with ADHD. Going to family outings, an amusement park, out to eat, or other activities can also seem overwhelming. Parents will try to avoid these activities with their child with ADHD or split the parenting. One parent takes the other children while one parent stays home with the "problem child." Neither solution works well. They both result in the child feeling like a "problem" or a "bother" and resentment from siblings.

When planning a public event or activity, it is important to know how to help the child plan for it. Advance discussions and, in some cases, role-playing can help the child know what to expect, know what is expected of him/her, and allows them to have confidence in their ability to handle the situation.

Children with ADHD do best when they know what to expect. Telling them specific times and possibly the schedule of events allows them to understand what is going to happen. Potential problems and changes in schedule can also be discussed with the child. It is essential to give the child the sense that there is structure, but also prepare them some events are outside of the parents' control. So, the structure may have to change.

This information should be given to the child in several ways. The initial presentation can be done verbally. It is important to remember to provide short, concise statements while having the child make eye contact, and then paraphrase back. This ensures the information was received and processed. The information can then also be given to the child in written form. Finally, for children who have smart devices, i.e., phones, tablets, laptops, the information can be placed in a scheduling app. Depending on the outing, the family can also role-play at home before going.

As with the house rules, it is vital to set up ahead of time what the ground rules are for any outing. This can be practiced on simple shopping trips by discussing with the child their ground rules before the shopping. Rules should be stated in short, direct sentences that state what the child is to do. For example, "You will stay by my side while in the store."

It is important to state the rules as things to do whenever possible. "Please keep your hands in your pockets," opposed to "Do not touch." Children with ADHD often do not process the word not and hear, "Do touch." Rewards and consequences should also be stated. Remember to keep rewards and consequences relevant. It will not work if you tell the child you will place them in time out if you do not have a way to do this or are not willing to do this at the store.

It is important to express confidence in the child when discussing the outing. Parents that convey they believe their child will succeed give the child confidence. This increases the child's belief in his/herself. It also decreases the child's anxiety. Reducing the emotions and the stress makes it more likely the child will be able to follow through with the rules.

The last important thing is managing time and experiences. All children have their limits on how long they can sit, pay attention, or passively watch something. Children with ADHD just have shorter limits. A child with ADHD needs to learn how to expand the time they can do these things, but that takes time and practice. It is helpful to start with shorter events and gradually build to larger ones. In this way, the child's success can help them increase their ability to control impulses in public.

Chapter 9: Causes Of Adhd

The exact reasons of ADHD are still unknown though scientists believe it is caused by an interaction between environmental or genetic factors with genetics playing a major role. Recent studies involving twins suggest that ADHD might run in families and 75% of cases are determined by genetics.

Genetic factors can also determine if ADHD can persist into adulthood. It is believed that people suffering from ADHD have low levels of Dopamine neurotransmitters.

It is predicted that the genes that control the levels or functioning of neurotransmitters (certain chemicals in the brain) are different in people suffering from ADHD. Knowing which genes cause ADHD can go a long way in minimizing the risk of manifestation of this disorder. Scientists are still conducting research to find ways to minimize the risks and factors associated with ADHD and reduce the chances of getting ADHD.

Be a role model for your kids – If you lose your temper in front of your child, take time to cool off and try to demonstrate self- calming techniques to teach your child to manage emotions in a better way. Don't shy away from apologizing to your kid.

In the event that a person is diagnosed with ADHD, the association abilities learnt during therapy will serve well later on. Indeed, even individuals who don't have ADHD discover they have to create these abilities before they take off to school or begin an occupation. Treatment for grown-up ADHD is like treatment for youth ADHD, and incorporates stimulant medications or different solutions, mental advising (psychotherapy), and treatment for any mental well-being conditions that happen alongside grown-up ADHD.

Many adults suffering from ADHD experience that they are often unpredictable and tend to forget appointments, miss important deadlines, and tend to make impulsive or irrational decisions. These behaviours can strain relationships and cause trouble in professional and personal lives.

As it might be overwhelming and frustrating to deal with a child suffering from ADHD, so it could be frustrating for the child to know that they are different. It is important for the entire family to accept this disorder as a part of life and make the best of it instead of focusing on the negative. The best way is to stay calm, celebrating life and giving your child the chance to make wise choices. Don't let ADHD become an excuse for bad behaviour, children must be taught to take responsibility of their actions and learn self-control.

If household routine gets too much to handle, it is suggested to get a pet. Although it might be a reluctant decision but having pets around can benefit both parents and children. Having a pet can make the child more responsible and channel-ize their energy in a better way. A pet can help the entire family in having fun and blowing off some steam. Various studies suggest pets can help in preventing depression, medical problems and stress.

It's difficult for ADHD affected children to learn social skills and mannerisms. Parents can teach children to become better listeners, understand body language, reading people's faces and interact properly in groups. Parents must discuss the problems and challenges their child might face honestly and teach them to make changes.

Strategies could involve role-playing various social scenarios, selecting playmates with similar language and physical skills, having zero tolerance for any physical act like hitting, pushing or yelling, rewarding good behaviour, making time and space to play, inviting more than two people at a time and observing their behaviour while they play.

Additionally, scientists believe other factors could also cause ADHD like:

1. Brain injury
2. Environmental factors like exposure to abnormal levels of lead found in pipes apparatuses or old paint structures
3. Low birth weight or premature birth
4. Consumption of tobacco or alcohol during pregnancy.

Chapter 10: All About Adhd: Causes, Types, And Risk Factors

"Did I cause this?" "What did I do wrong, and how could I have prevented it?" These are the common questions parents have when they learn their child suffers from ADHD. While it is OK and even endearing to feel responsible for your child, do not fall into the trap of blaming yourself for the development of ADHD in your child: the exact cause of ADHD is unknown. However, research has suggested that a couple of factors may cause ADHD.

ADHD: Causes

Let us look at some of them below:

Genetics

According to research, ADHD has a tendency of running in families because of inherited genes that play a significant role in the development of the condition. Research has shown that children with ADHD are five times more likely to have parents or relatives who suffer from the condition.

As of now, researchers are still investigating different genes with one particular gene of extreme interest being dopamine, a chemical those suffering from ADHD seem to have lower levels of it in the brain.

Exposure to Environmental Toxicity

Researchers have established a link between mothers who consume alcohol or smoke tobacco during pregnancy and the development of ADHD in children. One of the toxic substances that contribute to the development of ADHD is lead. Lead associates with hyperactivity, a behavior common in ADHD patients. Lead can especially cause ADHD if the lead exposure is within the first three years of a child's development. Lead can come from a smoking mother or the walls of an old building painted with the ancient paint rich in lead.

Nicotine and alcohol are the other toxics that affect brain tissues development and have prolonged effects on children's behavior when exposure occurs. Nicotine causes hypoxia, a lack of oxygen and this only makes the situation worse.

Brain Injury

Medical research and science have hinted at brain injury being a possible cause of attention deficit disorder in children. Brain injury may occur because of two things; one is exposure to toxins, and the second is physical injury before or after birth.

Medical experts suggest that head injuries may play a part in causing ADHD in individuals previously not suffering from the condition. Most research points to damages to the frontal lobe as the reason for this.

Brain Function and Structure

ADHD is a medical disorder also caused by a couple of factors that affect how the brain functions and develops. Researchers have found differences between brains of those suffering from ADHD and those who do not suffer the affliction.

The Basal ganglia, cerebellum, frontal lobe, caudate nucleus are some of the brain parts that regulate behavior. Their functions include self-monitoring, motor control, inhabitation, planning, working memory, emotional and verbal regulation, maintaining, and changing mental set. When one of these functions such as inhabitation does not work, it affects other functions, which models an ADHD brain structure.

The structuring of the brain may lead to the development ADHD. For example, research has found out that the brain of children with ADHD may take two to three years longer to mature compared to the brain of children unaffected by the condition. Other studies further suggest that children suffering from ADHD may have a chemical imbalance of neurotransmitters in their brains.

Other Possible Causes

Medical research also mentions other numerous causes as playing a big role in the development of ADHD; these include:

Lower weight at child birth

A premature pregnancy especially one that occur before the 37th week

Medical researchers also speculate that smaller brain volumes may lead to ADHD.

Some medical practitioners also believe nutrition and food may lead to ADHD. They cite refined sugar as being responsible for a couple of abnormal behaviors adjacent to the development of ADHD in children.

As is common with many disorders, ADHD has different types. In the next section, we shall look at the different types of ADHD.

Types of ADHD

Before 1994, ADHD was attention deficit disorder (ADD). After 1994, the medical fraternity renamed ADD to ADHD and further broke it down into three subtypes with each subtype having its own behavioral patterns or symptoms.

Medics and researchers categorized ADHD symptoms into three:

(i) Inattention: This symptom suggests someone has poor concentration, gets distracted easily, and has poor organizational skills.

(ii) Impulsivity: This person likes taking risks and interrupting.

(iii) Hyperactivity: This person has difficulty staying still and is constantly fidgeting, talking, and seems to slow down.

The Three Types of ADHD

As indicated above, ADHD breaks down into three subtypes as follows

Predominantly Inattentive ADHD

This type of ADHD denotes individuals who show symptoms of inattention more than they show symptoms of impulsivity and hyperactivity. Individuals suffering from this type of ADHD might have problems with hyperactivity and impulse control issues. The only difference is that the above two are not their dominant characteristics. Individuals suffering from inattention show the following symptoms:

They get bored quickly

They have trouble listening

It's hard for them to focus on one task or playing activities

They have bad memories and tend to be forgetful of daily activities.

They tend to lose personal things like notebooks, pencils, or other items they need to complete a certain task

They have a huge problem with learning new information or organizing thoughts.

They have a tendency to make careless and easily avoidable mistakes

They move slowly to a point where they appear lethargic or as if they are daydreaming

They have problems processing information; they process information slowly and less accurately compared to other individuals.

They have problems following directions

They also avoid tasks that involve effort

According to research from National Resource Center on ADHD, girls are at a higher risk of this type of ADHD.

Hyperactive-Impulsive ADHD

Individuals suffering from this type of ADHD have symptoms of hyperactivity and impulsivity as their main character traits. Individuals afflicted with this type of ADHD might also display signs of inattention, which does not predominantly manifest as the symptoms below:

They have difficulty sitting still

They have trouble participating in quiet activities

They are impatient

They are mostly restless

They constantly fidget and squirm

They like playing and touching objects even when the objects are not required for a task

They mostly act out

They do not think about the consequences of their actions

They like interrupting using behaviors such as shouting out inappropriate comments and answers.

They are always on the go; as if they are motor driven

Children suffering from this type of ADHD often make learning difficult for themselves and other students by constantly disrupting the classroom.

Combination ADHD

This type of ADHD is unique. Individuals and children diagnosed with this type of ADHD do not predominantly show the symptoms of inattention or hyperactivity. Instead, they show a combination of at least six symptoms of inattention and hyperactivity ADHD (six symptoms from each).

Who Is At A Risk Of ADHD?

ADHD often starts from childhood and continues to develop through adolescence and into adulthood. Seven years is the average age at which this disorder starts developing.

Studies have shown that the number of children diagnosed with this condition is on an increase; unfortunately, there is no clear explanation why this is the case. This disorder has affected about 9% of American children aged between 13 and 18 years. It has also affected about 4.1% of American adults between the ages of 18 years and older (these statistics are yearly).

Research into the nature of ADHD has also concluded that boys are four times likely to suffer from ADHD.

Having cultivated a substantial ADHD understanding, let us move to ADHD diagnosis and treatment.

Chapter 11: Adhd For Parents

Most children with ADHD come with a parent or relative. ADHD is not caused by excessive screen time, poor parenting or too much sugar consumption. ADHD will improve when children receive medication, eat healthy food, get enough sleep and exercise and have parents who are compassionate and know how to respond to ADHD. In this chapter, we define the causes and the solution of ADHD as well that how you help your child to get rid of it

2.1 What Are the Causes of ADHD

It's unclear what causes ADHD's brain differences. There is strong evidence to suggest that ADHD is mostly hereditary. Most children with ADHD come with a parent or relative. ADHD is not caused by excessive screen time, poor parenting or too much sugar consumption. When children receive treatment, eat healthy food, get enough sleep and exercise and have support, ADHD can improve. The exact cause of attention deficit hyperactivity disorder is not fully understood, although it is believed to be responsible for a combination of factors:

Genetics:

ADHD appears to be operating inside communities. As a result, parents and siblings of children with ADHD are four to six times more likely than parents of a neuro-typical child to have/inherit it. No single gene was identified as having induced ADHD. Various genes are more likely to be involved; each is interacting extremely complicatedly with the environment. The outcome may be that members of the same family have different types of ADHD.

The Brain:

Most ADHD children don't have a history of brain injury or brain damage. Studies using brain scanning techniques, however, found that children with severe ADHD symptoms were more likely to have lower than regular activity in the brain's frontal lobes. There is a chemical imbalance in the front of the mind of children with ADHD, with a reduction of certain natural chemical messengers-dopamine and noradrenaline. It is assumed that the brain's executive function is under control which results in ADHD symptoms.

Environmental Factors:

Exposure to smoking, alcohol and drug abuse during pregnancy, premature birth (before the 37th week of pregnancy), low birth weight and 13 brain damage - increase the risk of ADHD in children. The evidence for many of these causes, however, is inconclusive, and more research is needed to determine if they actually contribute to the ADHD.

Helping a Child with ADHD:

Whether or not the signs of inattention, hyperactivity and impulsiveness in your child are triggered by ADHD may cause many problems if left untreated. Children who cannot concentrate and manage themselves can fail in school, experience constant difficulty, and find it difficult to get along or make friends with others. Such struggles and challenges can lead to low self-esteem, tension and stress for the entire family.

Yet care can make a marked difference in the symptoms of your infant. Your child can be useful in all areas of life, with the proper support. If your child struggles with ADHD-like symptoms, don't wait to seek professional help. Without a diagnosis of attention deficit disorder, you can treat the symptoms of hyperactivity, inattention and impulsivity in your child. Options to begin with include getting your child to treatment, implementing a better diet and exercise plan, and modifying the home environment to minimize distractions.

When you have an ADHD diagnosis, then you can work with the doctor, therapist, and school of your child to develop a customized treatment plan that fits their specific needs. Successful early care for ADHD includes behavioral therapy, parent education and training, social support, and school assistance. Medication may also be used; however, treatment of cognitive disorder should never be the primary focus of attention.

Common Misbeliefs

ADHD is no other term for a kid who is naughty.

ADHD is not caused by poor parenting, but poor behavioral management may increase problem behaviors and improve special management techniques.

Recent research does not support previous dietary theories which cause hyperactivity.

2.2 What Can Parents Do?

If your child is facing hyperactive, inattentive or impulsive type, it might take a lot of energy to get him or her to listen, complete a task or sit still. The constant monitoring can be annoying and frustrating. You may feel like your kid runs the show sometimes. There are steps you can follow to regain control of the situation while helping your child make the most of his or her abilities at the same time.

Although attention deficit disorder is not triggered by lousy parenting, useful parenting techniques can go a long way to fixing patterns of problems. Children with ADHD need structure, consistency, clear communication, rewards and behavioral consequences. We also need lots of love, encouragement and support.

Parents can do many things to reduce the signs and symptoms of ADHD without losing the natural energy, playfulness, and sense of wonder that is special in every kid.

Take Care Of Yourself So You Can Take Better Care Of Your Child:

Eat right, exercise, get enough sleep, find ways to reduce stress, and seek support from family and friends, as well as from the doctor and teachers of your child.

Set Guidelines and Stick to It:

Help your child stay focused and disciplined through observing daily routines, simplifying the schedule for your child and keeping your child active with healthy activities.

Set Simple Expectations:

Simplify the rules of behavior and clarify what will happen when they are obeyed or violated and proceed with a reward or a penalty each time.

Encourage Sleep and Exercise:

Physical activity increases attention and fosters brain development. Importantly, it also leads to better sleep for children with ADHD, which in turn will reduce the ADHD symptoms.

Help Your Child Eat Right:

To manage ADHD symptoms, schedule healthy regular meals or snacks every three hours and cut back on junk and sugary food.

Teach Your Child How to Make Friends:

Teach him or her to become a better listener, learn how to read people's expressions and body language, and communicate with others more easily.

Be Involved:

Learn regarding ADHD as much as you can. Monitor the medication prescribed by your child's health care provider. Keep the needed therapy appointments.

Offer Pharmaceutical Drugs Safely:

If your child is taking ADHD medication, please offer it at the time and dosage prescribed. Hold pharmaceutical items in a safe place.

Work with The School for Your Children:

If your child should have an IEP, ask the teachers. Check regularly with the teachers to find out how your child is doing. Work together to help your child make things perfect.

Discipline with Intent and Warmth:

Understand what approaches to parenting are best for an ADHD child and what can make ADHD worse. Have an open and positive conversation with your child about ADHD. Reflect on the strengths and positive qualities in your kid.

Talk to others for help and awareness:

Join an ADHD support group to get updates on medication and other details.

Award Your Child for Good Behavior:

For a certain amount of time, make a deal to focus on a particular task. This is much more complicated than it sounds as the job has to be completed with a little extra effort from the child and the reward has to be considered carefully. It is necessary to explain the information thoroughly and to put a visual reminder in a strategic position. The activities and incentives need to be periodically changed and addressed with the child to maintain interest and compliance. For example, Conduct- spending two hours are playing nicely with a sibling. Reward-with an adult having an extra special playtime of 15 minutes.

Keep Routines:

Kids with ADHD are happier, calmer and more secure when they know what to expect. Keeping schedules wherever possible, can be extremely helpful. Routine changes can often cause confusion and anxiety that may activate disruptive behavior. Inform your child as soon as possible if improvements are essential to help reduce the potential regression in practice.

Until Giving Instructions in Bite-Size:

Children with ADHD often have problems remembering instruction lists. We usually cope at any given time with just one or two instructions. Confirm that you have their attention and make sure they understand your question before giving directions. 18 Build trust by encouraging things they are successful at 19. To be sure that attention is paid, often you have to:

- Switch off the TV/radio/music (with careful consideration)
- Use the child's name
- politely hold their hands and face them softly (for young children)

- Approach from the front (for older children)
- Have eye contact
- Talk clearly without shouting.

Teach new necessary conduct by describing, illustrating and, probably, completing the task together first. Then let the child execute it independently.

Make Clear Rules:

Write down and agree with your spouse, business, and reasonable, consistent rules of the household and show them in a prominent position. Conflicting laws make a child confused and irritated. Focus on areas of behavior, which really matter to you and other family members. Any harmful or damaging acts like hitting, kicking, scratching, slapping, punching or any additional aggressive or verbally abusive conduct must have consequences. Examples of implications may be removing a favorite toy for a certain period of time, such as a computer console for the remainder of that day. On less critical issues, you can be more flexible and not waste effort, such as not placing an item away, knocking things over or minor disruptions. That sounds easy, but sometimes it can be challenging. Using natural consequences wherever possible, such as losing a reward if a child is not ready on time. Explain what will happen to your child if they misbehave and violate the rules. Keep sticking by law, never give up, and stop yelling, constant criticism and idle threats. Children will copy all actions, good and bad.

2.3 Maintain a Positive Attitude

Kids with ADHD frequently fall into a negative circle, which makes them feel bad about themselves and also leads to low self-esteem and resulting in behavioral regression. Aim to establish a right circle of praise, which will make them feel good about themselves and, in turn, help improve their behavior. Increase confidence in your child by supporting them in the things they are good at.

Explain how well your child is at the game. Tell them what to do and not what to do. Catch them being kind, and give immediate verbal praise. Good sentences to use to reinforce good behavior:

I'm so pleased with you because?

Was that good when you did?

Does that make me happy when you?

We have time to do that now as you were so helpful?

Well done, all of this you did alone.

17 Children with ADHD need more frequent, more urgent, more effective and clear-cut reinforcement. Aim at delivering genuine positive comments about their behavior/activities at least 10 times a day. Do this when possible, in front of others. Note, you might want to sit or play quietly, tidy up toys, or share a game with a sister or brother. We don't even note still good behavior at times. Positive backing up helps your child to try harder.

2.4 Be Willing to Make Small Compromises

Same sacrifices leave significant effect try to make little compromises for your children's. Give them space and try to avoid arguments.

Paying attention to your child, despite being negative, may be seen as a reward for the child and may encourage the child to repeat unwanted behaviors.

Don't be too emotional.

Be specific to each other.

Don't exaggerate.

Rest assured.

Short message replay may be needed.

Time-out and approach to carrot-and-stick.

The idea to take a break or time out is to let your child, and you calm down. If time out isn't working, the approach to carrot-and-stick may work. Say, for instance: "John, I want you to go to the chair now. You can watch TV tonight if you go now. If you don't go now, tonight there won't be a TV. It's your decision."

Techniques to Avoid Trouble:

If possible, avoid recognized causes.

Plan ahead, e.g. when feeding the baby, the older child might need a fun activity or be encouraged to do something to help. When your child is helpful, remember to lend praise.

Give specific time reminders for future changes, e.g.' Time for a bath in five minutes,' then 3 minutes, 2 minutes and 1 minute.

Give positive orders, such as' please pick up your coat and hang it up' instead of' leave no mess on the floor.'

Using count downs, for example' I'm going to count to three, and if you're still yelling, you're going to have to go to your corner time out.'

Be realistic. If shopping trips after school are particularly troublesome, arrange the shopping trip, if possible, when the child may be elsewhere.

The children with ADHD can speak rudely, offensively or stupidly. Children imitate adults, so they don't allow bad language in the presence of adults. Be aware at all times that disrespectful comments are not appropriate.

2.5 Believe in Your Child

Parents are always in need to believe in their children and what they are capable of. If we do not have that confidence in our own kids, then who is going to?

When a child knows and thinks their parents believe in them, it can make them feel they can do something. We, too, will be more willing to put more time into what they do.

We are all able to believe in others. Parents should aim to show consistent confidence in your child as self-esteem can be challenging to maintain. In today's society, motivation and affirmation are so important when you consider the knockbacks children can face on a regular basis.

Often school kids can be cruel and will try to make each other feel bad over anything from test scores to appearance. Anything that in some way unfavorably compares them to other people.

Teaching Children Self-Belief:

Life is competitive, so we need to help our kids stay healthy and believe in who they really are. Fathers you have to prove you find in your boy! We can do this by thinking about how well they're doing using positive language to motivate them to concentrate on what they're doing not what their peers are doing and perhaps even showing their accomplishments and awards on our kitchen walls to demonstrate their achievements.

Occasionally, when they do something that seems out of character, a parent's trust in their child will be questioned. When a parent's confidence in their child is rocked, they need to resurrect their child's optimistic feelings and thoughts and realize they are still the same person. We previously believed in them, and we can do it again. Thinking in them will once again bring them back on the path they followed because they feel our sense of trust and love for them.

Chapter 12: Adult Adhd Symptoms - Which Type Of Adhd Are You Facing?

The very phrase 'adult ADHD symptoms' might be enough to make someone shiver. Who wants to go down a road that might end up in a diagnosis, the pursuit of which could lead to some letters added to a medical file somewhere? Life's problems are rarely about shoving uncomfortable realities out of sight, however. By looking the possibility of having ADHD in the face, an individual will be taking the first steps to finding a solution to the difficulties adult ADHD symptoms present. It is important to recognize that while adult ADHD symptoms are quite common and characteristic across the board in terms of hyperactivity, inability to focus, impulsivity, the Diagnostic and Statistical Manual for Mental Disorders (DMS-IV-TR) recognizes that there are three distinct categories of ADHD. Therefore, it is important to become familiar with each of the three in order to determine which category the specific adult ADHD symptoms an individual is manifesting best falls into.

ADHD, Predominantly Hyperactive-Impulsive Type:

Hyperactive adults have incredible difficulty waiting, especially for desired outcomes or activities. They seem to be constantly "on-the-go" and working on this thing, that thing or doing a myriad projects all at once. Sitting still is extremely difficult, especially if the individual is not enjoying whatever it is they have to sit and listen to. Adults with ADHD predominantly hyperactive-impulsive type appear to be always restless and unsatisfied with their current activity. They always want to move onto the "next thing" and lack a sense of contentment or mindfulness.

ADHD, Predominantly Inattentive Type:

Individuals with ADHD, predominantly inattentive type will have adult ADHD symptoms that would best be described as having their "head in the clouds" or "out of touch with reality." Individuals with the predominantly inattentive type are consistently accused of not listening very well, losing focus, becoming easily distracted and just "going off into dreamland." They will often appear 'spacey', unfocused, not present or disinterested. Disorganization and clutter are consistently the norm for individuals with the predominantly inattentive type of ADHD.

ADHD, Combined Type:

As the name would suggest, individuals with ADHD combined type manifest adult ADHD symptoms from both of the categories, a mixture of hyperactive-impulsive and inattentiveness all at once.

WHAT ARE THE CAUSES OF ADHD?

Unfortunately, no single ADHD cause seems to fit all cases. Research has uncovered many variables as to what causes ADHD, from brain activity, brain chemistry, genetic predisposition, to brain structure, but no one can point to just one thing as THE cause for ADHD. To further confuse the issue, with the introduction of MRI (magnetic resonance imaging) and PET (positron emission tomography) it is being suggested that the cause of ADHD in children may well be brain volume that is slightly less than those without ADHD.

Since the 1940's, when ADHD was first recognized as a treatable disorder, scientists have been investigating many theories as to the cause of ADHD including environmental toxins, food allergies, nutritional deficiencies, and food additives.

There are factors appear to be particularly important to the occurrence of ADHD/ADD, but not necessarily causative:
- Otitis media (ear infections)
- Nutrient deficiency (allergies to artificial colors flavors, additives, diet) and
- Heavy metals

Ear Infections

A higher frequency of ear aches growing up appears to be more common in ADHD/ADD children. This doesn't appear to be a cause of ADHD but rather a companion condition. The addition of Echinacea sp as an herbal supplement has proven to be effective in alleviating ear aches and maintaining good inner ear health. In addition, adding a humidifier to the child's bedroom for night time use can also aid.

Prior to birth, the decision to breast feed as opposed to bottle feeding may also be a positive contributing factor to ear health later on, with the position of the feeding infant, and other physical factors being the important considerations.

Nutrient Deficiency

Virtually any nutrient deficiency can result in impaired brain function, with

Iron deficiency being the most common in American children.

Several clinical studies, while not identifying the cause of ADHD do indicate that the addition of nutritional supplements can IMPROVE mental function in school-aged children.

Food / Preservatives Allergies

The Feingold Hypothesis is a study that suggests food allergies as the major contributing factor to causing ADHD/ADD. A diet REMOVED of refined flour, sugars, foods with color additives and preservatives has been proven to show amazing behavior and learning changes in a very short time, suggesting that the cause of ADHD is indeed an allergic reaction.

WHAT CAUSES ADHD IN KIDS?

ADHD is a common term. Some of us, especially those with kids who aren't working up to their potential, use the term "ADHD" or "ADD" all the time. Usually we mean that our kid is being hyperactive and can't pay attention. Or our child is dreamy and never seems to know what's going on.

In addition to how often we use the terms, it also seems like every expert (and lots of non-experts) has their pet theory of what causes ADHD.

A few of these theories that have been blamed for "causing" ADHD include
- Poor diet and too much junk food
- Allergies to artificial coloring (and flavoring)
- Bad parents
- Traumatic Brain Injury
- Vaccinations
- Too much TV
- Too many video games
- School is boring
- School is too hard
- Learning disabilities
- Right-brain kid in a left-brain world
- Lead poisoning

None of the above "cause" ADHD but they can cause behavior that looks like ADHD. And many of these factors when corrected will help with both ADHD and ADHD-like behavior.

Sometimes it's hard to sort out. For example, children with what researchers thought was ADHD have been put on the Feingold Diet.

The Feingold diet promoters suggest that poor diet causes ADHD and a better diet will "cure" it. This somewhat complicated elimination diet does help lots of kids. In some children, it eliminates ADHD symptoms totally. In other kids curb the symptoms a lot. But that doesn't mean that bad diet caused ADHD.

Chapter 13: Adhd In A Nutshell

Attention Deficit/Hyperactivity Disorder (ADHD) has had many alternative labels, including attention deficit disorder (ADD), minimal brain dysfunction, hyperkinetic syndrome, and developmental hyperactivity. This syndrome appears in early childhood and may have a lifelong course. Research findings show a primary deficit in the ability to inhibit responding, to delay responding, or to tolerate externally imposed delays in behavior once a task is begun.

Children with ADHD do not see the value in working hard at school, and academic achievement is often below the child's measured Intelligence. Sustained mental effort tends to be inherently punishing. Conflict with parents and teachers is common. Compared to most individuals of the same age there is more variability in the ADHD person's behavior across situations and time. Classrooms and other group settings requiring sustained attention to task produce much more symptomatic behavior than one-to-one situations, novel settings, or situations in which the person receives frequent feedback or reinforcement.

There are very few diseases or disorders that are diagnosed in children and don't carry over into adulthood. ADHD or Attention deficit hyperactivity disorder is one of those disorders that is usually diagnosed early on in childhood and persists throughout the person's life. It is a myth that as we become adults ADHD just disappears or goes away. In most cases, the person will have some if not all the same symptoms in adulthood as they did in childhood. Even though diagnoses of ADHD in children have increased over the last decade, there are many cases that go undiagnosed. Some children are able to cope with mild symptoms and therefore they aren't diagnosed until later on in life. Either way, most adults who are diagnosed with ADHD have had some types of symptoms all their life.

For any parent, it is hard to accept that your child has a disease or disorder. Guilt, anger and frustration are normal reactions. However, denial plays another role in some parent's inability to determine their children's actions or rather symptoms. When parents, teachers, or adults dismiss their child's symptoms for typical childhood hyperactivity or distraction, they are missing a key part of caring for their child's welfare. Not all children experience all the symptoms of ADHD therefore parents may label their child as a troublemaker or dreamer if they show an inability to concentrate in school. However, even one symptom can lead to a diagnosis and should be taken seriously. Some kids may be able to compensate for their symptoms due to a higher intellectual level. As they age adulthood can exacerbate their symptoms due to increased responsibility, and a greater demand for organizational skills. Although diagnosis of this disorder in childhood, gives people more time to educate, learn and manage their ADHD, adult diagnosis requires the same education, support from family and friends and creativity to manage their symptoms.

While the symptoms of ADHD are similar in childhood and adult ADHD, their appearance presents itself quite differently. Every individual has a unique set of symptoms and not all symptoms are required to diagnosis this disorder. Poor concentration, hyperactivity, distractibility, impulsiveness, and restlessness are key characteristics of ADHD. Adult ADHD primary symptoms include trouble concentrating or hyper focus, disorganization and forgetfulness, impulsivity, emotional difficulties, and restlessness. Adults are much less likely to be hyperactive than children, however it is included in the symptomology. If left untreated and undiagnosed adult ADHD can lead to problems in all areas of life, physical, mental, work, financial, and relationships.

Chapter 14: Be Realistic

Be realistic about the time it will take you to do something. We have trouble focusing, so we will probably get side tracked. Make sure you give yourself ample time on a task. If a normal person takes an hour. You should give yourself at least an hour and a half. I would even go as far to say two hours to be safe.
I will include ways to stay on task in situations where there is a time limit. Such as work or school, later on in the book. You won't always need the full amount of time alloted. It is just nice to know you have it if you do need it. Always make sure you are using your time wisely. Don't use your alloted time to mess around and not focus on the task. Having ADHD is a constant battle that never really gets easier. We just get better at managing it.
I definitely feel that you can grow out of it. I think as our brains change and grow, and we get better at handling it. That at some

point it may just go away. Until then, we have to do everything we can to make our lives easier and manageable. Once you get into a routine it becomes much easier. All you have to do, is stick to these tips and truly take my advice.

You Will Never Be Perfect

Tell yourself right now, that you will never be perfect. No matter how hard we try. It just will not happen. You may have perfect time management. You may keep lists of all the things you have to do. At one point or another you will forget or lose focus. That is perfectly ok and you should be ok with that. No one is perfect all the time. All we can do is try our best.

Put your best foot forward and take things one step at a time. It becomes really easy to beat yourself up and shut down when you are having trouble focusing. One thing we can't do is have a poor me attitude. The only thing we can do is keep moving forward and finding better ways to manage our brain. You will slip up and lose focus. You will have a bad day now and again.

You may make a mistake at work that costs you. But at the end of the day you have to stay focused and keep to your routine. As long as you stick to your personal routine you can't go wrong. Don't let anyone make you lose focus on your routine. They will understand if they have to wait on you.

Prepare Your Environment

Make sure your workspace, home, car or wherever you are is organized. I know it's tough to stay organized. But it is mandatory for someone with ADHD. You can set up a daily routine of tidying up around the house so it doesn't get overwhelming. This also can be done for making sure you don't forget anything. Such as a routine where you check appliances or make sure everything is in your pockets before you leave the house.

Try to have a quiet place to work and to focus. A room without a tv and no distractions. If you dont have a quiet room get some headphones and play ambient noise. You aren't stupid for not being able to focus with a lot going on. We just have to take extra steps to make sure we can stay focused and not get off track. Whatever it takes for you to stay focused is what you should do.

Everyone is different with their routines and the way they do things. You have to find the one that works for you. This is just a rough guideline for you to make your own. Through trial and error you will find the best way to keep focused and get the things you need to done.

Chapter 15: Treatment Options

Generally, the first line of treatment for ADHD suffers is medications. These medications are designed to help ADHD suffers concentrate and to limit their impulsiveness. The medications prescribed for ADHD most commonly are psychostimulants. These medications are considered controlled medications meaning you must have a valid and current prescription, and refills are tightly controlled. The most widely used stimulant medications are:

Ritalin
Adderall
Concerta
Daytrana
Focalin
Metadate CD
Dextrostat
Dexetrine

These medications are designed to stimulate the brain's production of certain neurotransmitters that seem to activate or turn on the attention and impulse control centers in the brain. They assist the brain on focusing the child's attention and to curb the impulsivity and hyperactivity associated with ADHD. These stimulant medications can have significant side effects however, and as such should be used in a controlled and closely monitored environment. The common side effects are headache, insomnia and loss of appetite. There are other, non-stimulant approved drugs for the treatment of ADHD. While not as effective, these medications are used if the side effects of stimulant medications are troublesome or become excessive.

Some of the common non-stimulant medications are:

Wellbutrin

Kapvay

Intuniv

Strattera

In addition to medications, a variety of behavioral methods have proven to be successful in managing the symptoms of ADHD. In the case of children, parent-child interaction therapy, which teaches parents how to bring out the desired behaviors while minimizing the inattentive or impulsive ones, is often used effectively. Parental training is another method that uses the parent to acknowledge and address the symptoms, and then, once the child is old enough, cognitive behavioral therapy teaches a child to control his or her behaviors by understanding how their thoughts and feelings are influencing them. Consultations with your child's teachers can help them better succeed at school, despite his or her disorder. Tools such as a daily reports that target desired behaviors have shown to be effective. Training in social skills may also help the child behave more appropriately with other children, and family group therapies can help parents and siblings manage the challenges created by the child's needs and behaviors.

Many children tend to outgrow their symptoms by the time they reach the middle school years, as symptoms begin to fade or disappear. Others however can continue to have symptoms that can seriously impair them as adults. Inattentive symptoms tend to continue into adulthood rather than hyperactive or impulsive. Many adults who still exhibit the inattentive symptoms tend to continue their medications and therapies throughout their adulthood.

Parents will frequently ask the following questions as their child or children are diagnosed with ADHD:

Did I do a bad job as a parent causing ADHD in my child?

No. ADHD is the result of chemical imbalances located within the brain, specifically in the area of the frontal lobe. A disorganized or abusive life at home can make it more difficult for children to deal with the symptoms of their disorder, and can result in even more impulsiveness.

Will my child outgrow ADHD?

Many children will eventually outgrow the original diagnosis, however symptoms can persist into adulthood, which will require them to continue to need professional help to manage them.

Will medications negatively affect my child's brain?

Based on studies performed on ADHD suffers, most of the medications used to treat ADHD have no long term effects on the structures of the brain. Children have been safely be on stimulant medications for years, however, as with any medications, you should always monitor them for any side effects that may be affecting them adversely.

Will medication affect my child's learning experience?

It Can. ADHD kids on medications tend to be able to concentrate more and are able to make the most of their time at school than before.

Will diet help with the ADHD?

While there is no scientific evidence as of yet to link the effects of diet and ADHD, diet can play a role with any behavioral conditions in children and adults. Some studies have recently shown that fish oil may help slow down symptoms of ADHD. The studies show that ADHD patients that use fish oils sometimes have more relief than those on Adderall, Ritalin, and other medications that are often given to ADHD suffers.

Some foods and beverages can have an adverse effect or enhance the symptoms of ADHD. Stimulant drinks such as coffee, sodas and even some fruit juices that contain excessive sugars or stimulants such as caffeine should be limited or avoided. Foods that contain excessive sweets or artificial ingredients can also make hyperactivity more prominent. Recent studies have also found that stimulants can cause some of the behavioral problems in both children and adults. Ritalin and Adderall, as well as other stimulating drugs have been linked to psychosis, bipolar conditions, manic depression, and schizophrenia episodes. More studies determining the link to diet and the effect on mental disorders such as ADHD are currently being performed.

Are the brains of ADHD suffers different than others?

Yes. Brain scans tend to show a difference in volume of the brain areas that focus on the attention and impulse control centers.

Chapter 16: Introduction: What Is Adhd?

Children who have trouble paying attention or find it hard to control his or her behavior might be suffering from attention deficit hyperactivity disorder or ADHD.

ADHD is a common type of mental disorder that affects children and may continue into adulthood. A person suffering from ADHD finds it hard to focus or concentrate, talks without a break and find it hard to stay still.

A child suffering from ADHD shows increased levels of inattention, impulsive behavior and hyperactivity than the other children of the same age. This affects their school performance and behavior at home. Fortunately, with the guidance of an experienced doctor and other specialists, this condition can be controlled to a large extent.

In this chapter, you will examine some of the causes of ADHD in children and the early symptoms that you must recognize as a parent. In addition, you will also explore some of the real life challenges you or your child are likely to face due to the condition.

What are the common causes of ADHD?

Unfortunately, there are no known factors that can cause ADHD. However, a majority of researchers believe that it occurs because of the complex interaction between our genes and the non-genetic or environmental factors.

Genetics is thought to play the most important role in causing ADHD. The disorder is believed to run in families with different genes playing a small role in the condition. Despite several theories, a genetic test is not yet available for diagnosing the disorder.

Some of the non-genetic factors that may cause ADHD in children include:

Low birth weight

Birth complications

Smoking or alcohol consumption during pregnancy

Exposure to toxic substances such as lead

Social deprivation

Neglect and abuse

Food additives and dyes that worsen hyperactivity

What are the early warning symptoms of ADHD?

ADHD has numerous symptoms. Some of these symptoms may seem like a normal behavior in the child at first, but those symptoms worsen over a period of time. A child suffering from ADHD shows at least six of the following symptoms related to inattention, hyperactivity and impulsiveness during the first 12 years of his or her life.

Inattention:

Does not seem to listen when spoken to

Habit of daydreaming and gets confused easily

Become bored with a task easily until something interesting is given to them

Gets distracted easily and misses out on important details
Cannot focus on more than one thing simultaneously
Finds it hard to organize or complete a task
Not able to learn anything new
Not able to follow the instructions
Processes information slowly and less accurately as compared to others

Hyperactivity
Talk non-stop
Not able to sit still in school or at home
Constantly remains in motion
Touches or plays with anything that comes into sight
Wriggles or twists their body in his seat
Feels difficulty in doing any task quietly

Impulsivity
Feels impatient
Finds it difficult to wait for the things they want
Spontaneous blur of words and emotions
Acts without thinking about consequences

Interrupts others' conversations and activities

Sometimes, it is difficult for you, as a parent, to identify the ADHD symptoms in your children that need immediate attention because the symptoms may look like other behavioral problems that are common in the kids at this age like lack of interest in studies, unwilling to listen to the parents or anger issues. For example, when a child sits quietly in a corner, you may think that he or she is doing the homework; though in fact it could be a sign of anxiety due to the inability to follow the instructions. Or you might mistake the hyperactivity or bad behavior at school with the disciplinary or emotional problems.

In case, you have been observing your child having trouble in adjusting with others or following the normal daily activities at home or school for a long time, you should immediately consult a doctor as these symptoms could be due to ADHD.

The types of ADHD

ADHD can be categorized into three subtypes as described below:

(1) Predominantly hyperactive-impulsive type: **The symptoms of this type mostly belong to the hyperactivity-impulsivity categories.** Inattention might be present despite the presence of less than six symptoms.

(2) Predominantly inattentive type: A majority of symptoms belongs to the inattention category. Hyperactivity-impulsivity may still be present despite showing fewer than six symptoms. A child suffering from the predominantly inattentive type of ADHD gets along well with the other children. They may sit quietly and not pay attention to anything; thus, there are chances that you might overlook them and not notice ADHD.

(3) Combined inattentive and hyperactive-impulsive type: Such children show six or

more symptoms from all the categories. A majority of children have this type of ADHD.

Challenges associated with ADHD

Children and teens with ADHD can have a tough time managing their school and personal life. Even though hyperactivity gets better as the child becomes a teen, problems like disorganization, inattention and poor impulse control may continue.

Such children may find it difficult to concentrate in school and hyperactivity may cause an increase in the behavior-related complaints from the school. As the child reaches the teenage, the risky behavior and not following the rules and regulations may become a major hindrance in achieving their educational and career goals.

A majority of adults with ADHD does not know that they suffer from it. A typical adult suffering from ADHD may have a history of failure at home or problems at work. It is difficult for them to stick to a single job, arriving on time at work and be productive.

In case, you or your child suffers from ADHD, there are a number of steps you can take to minimize its effect on your daily activities and also help your child overcome the challenges. You will read about these steps in the coming chapters. The purpose of this book is to provide guidance to the ADHD-affected adults and the parents of the children suffering from the disease so that they are able to overcome the obstacles created by the same in the personal, professional, social and academic spheres of their life. Read on to know how you can begin your journey towards an independent adulthood in spite of having ADHD.

Chapter 17: Understanding Adhd's Impact

One of the most important things that you as a parent need to understand about your child with ADHD is that their brain functions differently than everybody else's. However, just because their brains function differently doesn't mean that they can't be taught how to behave, it is just that you are going to have to do things a bit differently. Children with ADHD have problems with impulse control; they often do things without thinking through the consequences of their actions. Dealing with impulsive children can be quite exhausting, but if you understand the impact that ADHD has on them and your family it can make things easier.

Children diagnosed with ADHD have a very hard time adapting to the social norms, those behaviors that we expect from children. They struggle in the real world because they lack the ability to plan ahead, and for these children it is what is happening right now that demands their focus. Children with ADHD have a hard time focusing on a single thing, they are easily distracted. Being easily distracted makes it hard to complete things that are required from the children, both in school and at home.

Many parents tend to think that children with ADHD are flat out ignoring what they are being told to do, while school mates and even parents think that these kids are just being plain annoying. Their behavior is often considered embarrassing when out in public, where society expects all kids to act a specific way. What you need to understand as a parent is that your child is not acting this way deliberately; they simply have no control over their behavior. If it was up to them they would sit quietly in the restaurant, they would do what they were told the first time or at least the second time. These kids want to do what is asked of them, but their ADHD prevents them from knowing how to do this.

When it comes to parenting a child with ADHD you not only need to understand the impact ADHD has on your child, you must also understand the impact it can have on your entire family. As you have probably already discovered the behaviors can cause a total disruption in your family's life. One of the biggest problems caused by their behaviors is that they don't "listen" to your instructions, so they don't do what they are told. Children with ADHD are easily distracted, which can create problems when you are in a hurry or are simply getting ready to go somewhere. Being easily distracted often causes them to lose track of what they were supposed to be doing, so the entire family ends up waiting on them and can even be late to important events.

If you have more than one child, parenting a child with ADHD becomes even harder. If you are not careful your child's siblings can end up resenting or even feeling jealous of the child with ADHD. Siblings often feel this way because children with ADHD often demand attention and won't stop until they get what they want. Their siblings are not as outspoken or demanding, so are easily overlooked. Parenting children with ADHD takes up a lot of time and energy, but it is vital that you don't overlook or take your other children for granted.

Perhaps the biggest impact is on the parents themselves. At the end of a long and especially tiring day you are going to find yourself both physically and mentally exhausted. Parenting a child with ADHD involves near constant supervision, not to mention the constant repeating of instructions and the pleas to slow down. Parenting a child with ADHD can be extremely stressful, but it is even more difficult when you don't understand their behaviors.

Rather than become frustrated and angry at your child's behaviors, accept the fact that they cannot control these things. Being frustrated and angry is never fun, for either you or your child. Learning behavior management therapy can help you successfully parent your child with ADHD.

Chapter 18: Attention: Deficit Or Surplus?

When we think about someone with ADHD, we usually think about someone who is easily distracted, forgetful, fidgety and unable to finish their work. In fact, a high level of distractibility is one of the key indicators of ADHD. But distractibility is only part of the ADHD story.

The same kid who can't get his math homework can play video games for hours. The adult who can't get his work done can spend hours surfing the net or watching TV. If getting distracted is part of having ADHD, how is it that these individuals can stay focused on certain things but not others? This is a common question heard in the therapist's or doctor's office. If they can focus on the things they like, do they really even have ADHD? The answer is YES but not in the way you might think!

Hyperfocus in ADHD

It turns out, the term "attention deficit hyperactivity disorder" is somewhat inaccurate. ADHD is not a **deficit** of attention at all but rather an **abundance** of attention. The problem is regulation of that attention. People with ADHD have problems shifting attention from one task to another. This phenomenon is frequently referred to as "hyperfocus" or "persistence."

Hyperfocusing is that uninterrupted laser-sharp attention on certain activities often to the exclusion of other sometimes very important things. Not surprising, these activities tend to be the ones we are most interested in and challenged by. When a person with ADHD is really interested in something, they can become laser focused and perform with stellar results. If they're not interested in the activity, then attention will start to wander and very little will get done. (Kimball, 2013). The challenge for a person with ADHD is how to regulate that attention so that the not fun tasks can get done along with the fun things they enjoy most.

So why does hyperfocus happen? Neuropsychological research suggests that abnormally low levels of the neurotransmitter dopamine in the brain's frontal lobes may affect attention and distractibility (Blum et al., 2008). This dopamine deficiency affects the brain's reward center and makes it hard to switch from one task to another, especially if one task is really interesting and the other is boring or undesirable.

Most people can shift from a highly desirable task to a less desirable one fairly easily. We don't like it but it's relatively easy. For people with ADHD, it's harder to make that shift. So, if little Johnny loves video games, when mom says, "It's time for dinner,", little Johnny's brain barely registers the information and remains focused on the video game in front of him. Mom is frustrated. Johnny is in trouble for not getting off of his game. Interestingly, the same phenomenon would be present if Johnny loved doing math problems. If his object of focus was math problems, his mom would still have the same issue of getting his attention away from the math and on to coming to dinner.

Hyperfocus, persistence, flow...whatever you call it, is neither good nor bad. The inability to focus on boring tasks is the same attention that propels people forward to excel at the things they love. The key is learning to regulate that attention and harness it in ways that are most productive for the person.

Executive Functioning and ADHD

A discussion about ADHD would not be complete without recognizing the role of executive functioning (EF). EF and "self-regulation" have become popular terms in the ADHD literature. ADHD is characterized by problems of self-regulation. Self-regulation is just that. It is the ability to monitor and manage one's behavior appropriate to the situation. Reading quietly in the library and not singing your favorite song because we are supposed to be quiet in a library. Not turning flips in your chair in class because the rule is that you sit in your seat. Basically, it is making behavior choices that are appropriate for the setting.

In its simplest terms, EF is a specific kind of self-regulation skills that helps people get things done. It's kind of the "boss" part of the brain – the frontal lobe - that gets things done. In people with ADHD, their frontal lobe is under-stimulated so they have difficulty monitoring their behavior. EF plays a significant part in time management, attention and problem-solving – all problems associated with ADHD. So, part of treating ADHD is improving EF and self-regulation.

Chapter 19: Treatment Through Lifestyle Changes And Habits

Despite the prevalence of ADHD, it is complex, with cases varying from child to child. For this reason, it's difficult to provide tips and recommendations that will work for each and every child. However, the suggestions, remedies, and parenting tactics outlined in this chapter are fairly universal and applicable to most ADHD cases. Some of the following focuses on creating an environment in which a child who has ADHD can succeed.

Remember, it's important to work in harmony with your child's teacher and principal as he spends a good deal of time at school. Talk to his school about making the necessary accommodations to better serve your child's needs. Your child will be able to accomplish his goals when he has the right tools, treatment, and support.

Show a lot of affection. Children who have ADHD need to be assured that they are loved and appreciated. Putting too much focus on the negative aspects of your child's condition such as bad behavior is counterproductive. Doing so will work against your treatment plan by harming the relationship between parent and child. Your child's self-esteem and self-confidence will be wounded as well.

Due to his symptoms, your child may find it difficult to recognize and accept verbal signs of affection. In this case, find other methods of showing affection. Give your child a hug, a pat on the back, or a simple thumbs-up to encourage him. Keep an eye out for behaviors that may call for compliments.

2. **Learn acceptance and give due attention.** It is important to accept both the negative and positive aspects of your child's personality. It is just as important for your child to know he is accepted despite his condition. Make an honest effort at spending more quality time with your child where no other adults or

children can interfere. This will enable you to give your child the positive attention he needs to stick with his treatment plan.

3. **Increase your child's self-esteem and build a sense of discipline.** Self-esteem is your child's armor against the challenges of ADHD. Find ways to build up your child's self-esteem. Try getting your child into karate, dance lessons, or martial arts classes—but never force your child into activities. Such activities will gradually build a sense of discipline in your child. ADHD children who know their strengths and weaknesses will naturally develop a high self-esteem. These children tend to have a better handle on the ADHD life and dealing with conflicts and negativity.

4. **When giving directions, use simple words.** Children with ADHD have difficulty following instructions. They can't help it, but you can. Whenever you give your child instructions, make sure to speak slowly, and be very specific and concise. Make eye contact while you are giving directions. It

is important to work with the symptoms of ADHD, and give foolproof instructions that are easy for your child to follow

5. **Help your child develop organizational skills.** Always keep your child's room neat, minimalistic, and organized. This way, he will have an example to refer to while the two of you work on developing his organizational skills. Make use of a daily assignment notebook. Consider grouping the objects in your home according to class, and mark them off with one- or two-word labels.

It is possible to wean your child out of the habit of clutter. You can even make a game out of it at the grocery store or local mall. Point out the aisle reserved solely for drinks or the shoe section. Be creative when teaching your child organization, and put elements of fun into the routine so as to prevent boredom. Furthermore, be sure to provide an environment that remains continuously uncluttered for your child.

6. **Keep a regular schedule for meals, naps, and bedtime.** Set a fixed time for meals, snacks, naps, and bedtime. Get your child into a routine; eventually, he will learn to follow that routine on his own. Keep in mind, however, that children with ADHD have a difficult time adjusting to sudden change, so find a way to break it to them gently. Consider making gradual, instead of sudden changes. For one week, get him into the habit of sleeping at a certain time. Then, the following week, work on a new habit, like snack time, and so on and so forth.

7. **Ensure your child gets proper rest.** Fatigue is known to worsen ADHD symptoms. Avoid overtiredness in your child by conditioning him to go to sleep and wake up at the same time every day. Because children with ADHD are often hyperactive, and spend a lot of time on the go, it is important to allow them naps during midday.

8. **Monitor your child's diet.** Your child's diet may or may not affect his ADHD symptoms, but it's important to know the effects of certain dietary habits. Good nutrition can actually make a huge difference by improving ADHD symptoms.

Keep your child on a regular meal and snack schedule, with each meal being no more than three hours apart. Doing so will help control your child's blood-sugar levels, decrease irritability, and promote concentration. Try to incorporate proteins and complex carbs into each meal as doing so will minimize hyperactivity. Omega-3 fatty acids are also helpful as they can aid in curbing hyperactivity and impulsiveness. Also, consider having your child take a daily multivitamin that contains zinc, iron, and magnesium.

9. **Learn to identify potentially difficult situations.** The lives of children who have ADHD should be simplified whenever possible. Avoid bringing your child into difficult situations such as movie theaters

and churches where he is required to sit down for long periods of time. A simple trip to the supermarket can be difficult due to the wide array of products that may overwhelm your child. Don't completely eliminate trips to the store or shopping malls as doing so is akin to erasing the fun out of his life. Rather, decrease the frequency of such trips.

10. **Be patient.** "Patience is a virtue." The old saying is especially true when you have a child who suffers from ADHD. Frustration is normal for parents, so don't feel bad. Consider practicing relaxation techniques whenever you find your patience wearing thin. Deep breathing, meditation, and visualization are a few options. Never show your child impatience as doing so will only discourage him. Even if your child's symptoms are so severe that he's out of control, it's imperative to remain calm. Doing so is model behavior that your child is likely to adopt as well.

11. **Use proper consequences when disciplining your child.** Discipline is an essential part of your child's treatment plan as it fosters good behavior. Consistent discipline teaches a child what behaviors are acceptable and unacceptable. The main goal of discipline in an ADHD treatment plan for children is to defuse out of control behavior. Teaching your child discipline will train your child to accept the consequences of his actions and choices. In the long run, your child will be respectful, happy, and able to find his place in the world as a well-behaved adult. Timeouts are a timeless method of discipline. Keep timeouts short, but long enough for your child to regain control.

12. **Implement a system of rewards for good behavior.** Getting out of the habit of behaving badly is only possible when incentives are put in place. Reward your child for a job well done, finishing his homework, or putting away his toys.

Children love praises. Rewards may come in the form of ice cream, a trip to a play park, or putting a quarter into your child's piggy bank.

13. **Be honest with your child about his condition.** If your child is old enough to understand, that is. Explain ADHD in simple terms. When a child knows exactly what is going on, he will likely exhibit better behavior in order to "conform."

14. **Don't allow your child to make ADHD an excuse.** When a child knows he has ADHD, he will use that knowledge as a convenient excuse. Don't treat your child too differently from his siblings or friends.

15. **Avoid overprotecting your child.** Sure, ADHD children need a little more protecting than children with normal behavior. As your child progresses through the developmental stages, it is important to learn when to let go in order to teach him independence. Pick and choose the few battles you will fight for with your

child, but leave him to defend himself in most of his battles.

16. **Deal with bad behavior wisely.** Withhold privileges whenever your child behaves badly. Perhaps you can implement a three-strike system, and only use punishment on the third strike. Whatever punishment you decide to use, make sure it's not too extreme. Some options may include withholding video games for half a day or TV time.

17. **Make to-do lists.** Keep your child on track by making a clear list of assignments and chores that your child needs to do. Use a dry-erase or chalk board that you can attach to your refrigerator. Make sure your handwriting is neat, and be very specific. To-do lists can help your child follow instructions more easily.

18. **Give your child bite-sized projects.** Doing so will help him develop organizational skills and improve his ability to follow directions. For instance, instead of telling your child to do his homework,

be specific and tell him to finish his math assignment. Then, write up a 5-question worksheet based on his math assignment for him to complete. Another tiny project you can give your child is a short book review. Have him read a short book, then write 3-5 sentences about what he learned.

19. **Eliminate distractions.** Don't let your child fall victim to his symptom of distractibility. Instead, make things easier for him. Cut down on distractions at home by turning off the TV, radio, and closing the living room blinds. This is especially recommended during homework and study time. Work with your child's teacher, and have him or her move your child's seat away from the window. Perhaps it would be best to have your child sit closer to the front of the classroom, directly in front of the board.

20. **Develop a relationship with your child's teachers.** Schoolteachers act as parents in your stead during school hours.

For this reason, it's important for your child's teachers to be aware of his condition. Stay in close communication with teachers and ask them to monitor your child's work, be flexible, and provide feedback. Teachers don't need to give children with ADHD any special treatment, however, giving clear instructions is important for those children to succeed in school.

21. **Ask about school programs.** By law, schools are required to have special programs for children with learning disabilities. Take advantage of any ADHD programs that your child's school offers.

Chapter 20: Helping Children With Adhd

Setting up a behavior modification program for children with ADHD takes hard work, commitment, devotion and collaboration between teachers, parents and caregivers. Behavioral management is a great spot to begin in just about any treatment plan that is complete. It includes learning new skills which can include impulse control, problem solving, anger control, and communication. The best results happen when everyone takes part in the training. There are there are only three kinds of behavioral therapy to take into account, these consist of positive reinforcement, social skills training, and cognitive behavioral therapy.

Cognitive refers to how you think about yourself and situations you end up in and of course the behavioral part refers to how you act. Cognitive Behavioral Therapy is devised by helping the child learn self-control by thinking before responding.

Typically, people with ADHD lack an internal voice that helps them control their whims. CBT can retrain the way your child behaves, thinks and acts.

Social skills training teaches children how to stay focused while they're with others and control their conduct as well. It helps them learn to eventually become less aggressive and impulsive. Techniques include practicing means to settle conflicts, and watching video tapes of good conduct, role playing, coaching. These techniques help them become more aware of how they act and more to the point how their actions affect others. Kids in social skills training programs also find out how to listen and take part in conversation, enter new group scenarios, cope with frustration, and additionally give and get criticism and praise.

Positive reinforcement is a reward system used to encourage good behaviour. It especially works with children. Kids can learn the consequences of both nice and bad behaviour, with regular reward. This method is useful at home and in school. Establish a duplicate reward like a treat or a special privilege, and then the key to this aim is to get a goal for good behaviour.

Individual treatment is designed for a therapist to work close with the individual child. Goals that are measurable are targeted by it in a one on one setting to create a plan to promote positive changes in ones life. It helps in coping with depression and low self esteem, as well as supplies real plans establish priorities to help the child stay focused, and help them manage issues in their own lives.

Group therapy may also be useful for children with ADHD. In a group kids learn how to socialize with others. Group therapy options include family therapy, couples therapy, group therapy that is large and small group therapy. Group therapy may give your child a connection to a community of children going through the same issues, a sense of acceptance, and moral support.

Establish. Perfection must not be expected. You can be in a better position to supply the essential guidance through the issues of ADHD by seeing through your childs eyes. No one can handle the challenges of ADHD on their own particularly a child.

In conclusion, learning all you can about children with ADHD is the solution to receiving the specific situation under control. Children that have ADHD need good role models for good conduct more than other children. Be honest and consistent in your own behavior continuously.

Chapter 21: The "Few Foods" Diet

This diet is more difficult than the last one, because it restricts more of the aliments that your child usually eats, and requires lifestyle changes that are, to say the least, challenging.

You can call it an extended diet because you have to exclude all the things previously mentioned and some more.

The few foods diet excludes:

Wheat
Chocolate
Soy/tofu
Corn products
Milk
Eggs

This may sound drastic, but if you tried the Feingold diet and hasn't done the job quite as you expected, this could be the right answer for your family.

On this diet you must eliminate as many foods as possible, from the one listed.

By now, you are probably wandering what your child can eat. He or she can eat fresh meat, rice, as many veggies that you can convince them to eat, with the exception of corn, and they can drink fresh juice, but not from citrus fruit.

Assuring that they get enough nutrients will be hard, but on the bright side, the restrictions are limited because you are merely trying to identify the foods that cause problems, and after two weeks you can start adding ingredients, one at the time. When you add aliments you must have a waiting period of several days in which you wait and see if that particular food has caused a reaction. If no negative reaction is noticed you can add another food and so on. Don't forget to write down in the diary any changes that might appear.

We've talked about what to eliminate from the diet but, while reading this I'm sure that you were asking yourself why you should do that and which are the reasons for using such a restrictive diet.

There is a particular thing called food sensitivity. Although sensitivity sounds like an allergy or intolerance it is not the same thing. When faced with an allergy or intolerance to a certain food, one would expect a physical reaction. In the case of food sensitivity, the physical, evident response isn't there or, if it is, it isn't noticeable. Sometimes the food sensitivity can cause a rash or stomachaches even headaches, but the peculiar and important, response in the case of children suffering from ADHD, could be an increase in hyperactivity and a decrease in concentration, if the reaction is aggressive it could lead to impulsiveness and an aggressive behavior.

This is the case of many people and of many children, the condition affects adults and children alike and the sooner measures are taken, the better for everyone.

Sensitivity can be related to any food, sometimes to a group of foods, like in the case of gluten or casein sensitivity.

Gluten is found in cereals like wheat, rye and barley but in other items to. People suffering from Celiac disease can't eat it at all, but a sensitivity wouldn't come up in blood tests like it would with any disease.

Casein is found in milk products like yogurt, kefir, cheese and all the end products, which come from milk.

The list of aliments that could be responsible for your child's sensitivity could go on; this is why it's so important to try the few foods diet, in order to eliminate all the possibilities.

You probably noticed that wheat is on the top of the list. It is not found there just because it could trigger a gluten sensitivity reaction. Wheat contains a high amount of nutrients and it should be an important part of every healthy person's diet, but the nutrients contained are transformed into sugar very fast.

We already discussed how sugar is a negative element in the diet of a child suffering from ADHD so, you must understand that any foods that, when broken down by the digestive system, will be high in glucose, should be avoided.

Chapter 22: How I Influence My Child's Behavior

Children are learning machines. In fact, we all are. Their sole role in society is to learn their place in the world and adapt their behaviors to fit in those places. Therefore, to address ADHD without addressing the social dynamics surrounding a child is to do a disservice to them. Our children do not live in a vacuum, and so as we take a closer look at this disorder, it is important that we put it in proper perspective.

Of all the social dynamics that a child must learn to adapt to and fit in, the family is the most important. In most cases, the future success of a child with ADHD hinges on how the family responds to his needs. Because of the close interaction with parents, siblings, and others in the household, how well the child develops those missing executive skills can be impacted in major ways.

For that reason, diagnosing ADHD is not as important as how this fact will affect the family dynamics. A diagnosis does not determine how well treatment will be or how the child will overcome the challenges they face. And as parents are the primary caretakers, they will be the ones that have the most influence on the child's progress through the hurdles he has to face with ADHD. With that in mind, every parent must ask themselves how their reaction to their child's behavior will influence their progress.

This becomes a powerful psychological exercise that will not only reveal the weaknesses in your child but your own weaknesses. There is no secret that managing a child with ADHD is no picnic, without their ability to control emotions, follow through on certain tasks, or to even attain to a certain level of independence, the impact can bring out the worst in many of us, especially that of a busy parent.

So, ask yourself just how do you react when you're at your wit's end; when you have tried cajoling, negotiating, yelling, prompting, and bribing to no avail. It is important at this point that you be entirely truthful with yourself because your reaction may be a contributing factor in your child's ability to adjust to this particular disorder.

This chapter is designed to give you a bird's eye view of your family dynamics and how it may be affecting your child. The questions asked can be hard to accept, but if you are open and honest about the answers, you will reap the rewards in the end. Below is a list of questions you should take into consideration.

Are you married or are you a single parent? If married, is your relationship a positive one or do you allow the negative aspects to spill over onto your children? Do you see your spouse or partner as a source of support or is it the opposite?

Do you work outside the home? If so, is your job stressful and do you at times bring that stress home with you?

Does your work bring you professional satisfaction or does it drain you of your energy, leaving you unfulfilled?

How do the siblings interact with the ADHD child? How much of that interaction is monitored and regulated by you and what examples have you set for the rest of the family.

It cannot be overstressed that the family dynamics of a child with ADHD is critical in understanding the child and helping them to navigate the challenges they face. Not only do these interactions tend to be more stressful but evidence has shown that these interactions can have a huge impact on a child's psychological state as well. In fact, statistics show that since the disorder can be genetic, there is about a 25-40% chance that a child with ADHD also has a parent that is also dealing with the problem. This increases the problem exponentially for the entire family. Here is how it usually goes...

Parents who are already involved in personal problems see their child's behavior as an intrusion on their stressful lives. The ADHD child's disruptive tendencies are perceived as consuming their valuable time and demands too much from them.

Parents then react negatively to the child's conduct in the form of harsh punishments, emotional outbursts, and irritability.

Parents may also withdraw supportive words of encouragement, recognition for good behavior, and the normal warmth and love that every child needs.

The child then responds in kind, usually in defiance, stubbornness, or some other negative emotion or attitude.

The behavior is then reinforced in the parent's mind identifying the child as rebellious or a disruptive influence in the family.

The cycle then repeats

It becomes a circle that never ends. The parents are stressed and withdraw affections that the child needs. Then, the child responds to negative input negatively and the cycle repeats. This may occur over and over again throughout the child's lifetime spreading to all other members of the family as well. In the end, you have a family unit that is dysfunctional, and no one is happy.

This is not to say that the parent's actions are deliberate. In fact, many may not even realize that they are doing it, but it is up to the parents to stop the cycle and get the family on a more nurturing and positive track. This can be even much harder if the parent involved is also ADHD.

Difference Between Mother's and Father's Interactions with ADHD

Some parents comment that there is a difference in how a child with ADHD responds to their parents. Often mothers point out that they tend to have more difficulty with their children than the fathers do. There have been several studies done to determine how accurate this statement may be. One study did show that children tended to give more negative responses to mothers than they did with the fathers.

While the reason for this is unclear, there are a few theories that may explain this particular problem within the family dynamic. One primary theory is that in most families the mother is the primary caretaker and as she is trying to reign in the child's self-control and as a result, negative reactions tend to occur. She is more likely to engage in conflicts with the child than the father who takes a lesser role in the managing of ADHD skills.

Mothers also tend to use more verbal skills in reasoning with their child than fathers do. Since children with ADHD generally struggle with language expression, are less likely to respond to verbal guidance and less likely to absorb the instructions given and therefore will quickly get irritated. Fathers, on the other hand, are not usually the ones to spend a lot of time repeating instructions and may be quicker to punish when results are not met. Therefore, one may draw the conclusion that a parent who talks less and follows through quickly seems to be the one that the ADHD child is most likely to respond to.

Interactions Between ADHD Children and Their Siblings

Next, to the parents, the dynamics of the ADHD child with his siblings also need to be carefully analyzed. It is a known fact that children with ADHD are more likely to argue more, fight more, and even get into or encourage more improper behavior than those without. This will inevitably involve more conflicts in the household.

There is no question that it can be frustrating living your life with an ADHD child. It's no wonder that children without the disorder may feel put upon and treated unfairly. This could naturally lead to resentment from siblings in having to share an additional burden of responsibility in the household when they are expected to pick up the slack with chores that the ADHD child has yet to master. There may also be a measure of envy as they notice that the ADHD child gets more attention and help from the parents than they do.

All of these factors can serve as fuel for an already tense situation and if not handled in the right way could lead to major difficulties for everyone.

What Does it All Mean?

It all comes down to one simple fact, having anyone with ADHD in the home can be stressful, but it is even more stressful when it is a child. Living with ADHD impacts everyone in the household so treatment must also include everyone in the household. Dealing with ADHD is challenging in the best of situations, so it's important for everyone involved to recognize this from the start.

In Part II of this book, we'll give you a few guidelines that can make home life easier to deal with as you start your treatment plans for ADHD. The good news is that there is light at the end of the tunnel. If you can bear up under the inevitable levels of stress, you will have to face it will be that much more rewarding when you see your ADHD child grow up to find their place in the world and grow up to be a responsible adult.

Conclusion

It scares me when I look back on my life and see how many hours I have wasted by running around confused, either looking for things I could not find, or jumping between tasks I was originally supposed to do. I often think: what a waste of a life; a waste of resources and a waste of others people's resources and patience.

I hope that with this book and the techniques I have described, you will be well prepared for your journey towards a more bearable life with ADHD. I can only smile and be happy at the thought of what these techniques have taught me, and how it has changed my life for the better. For now I know that success is not only the entitlement of the resourceful. No, now you and I can also set our self goals and have high ambitions. We do not necessarily need to be slaves of our "disability". It's about taking responsibility for your own life and doing something. As long as the desire to achieve your objectives is big enough, there is nothing that can stop you!

If you received value from this book, I would like to ask you a favour. Would you be kind enough to leave a review on Amazon for this book. This is my first book and it's hard to get noticed as a new writer. You leaving a review will help me get more exposure for my book. I really want to reach as many people as I can and help them to improve their quality of life.

I wish you the best of luck on your journey towards a more efficient life.

CPSIA information can be obtained
at www.ICGtesting.com
Printed in the USA
LVHW081355050321
680689LV00032B/532